LIFE

RULES

A Manual to Attain Happiness

**Nine Basic Rules to Follow to Help you get
Peace of Mind in a Stressful World**

Deacon Robert W. McCormick

Deacon Robert W. McCormick
275 Main Street
Hornell, NY 14843
607-324-5880
rwmccormick@infoblvd.net or bob@infoblvd.net

Limits of Liability and Disclaimer of Warranty

The author and publisher shall not be liable for your misuse of this material. This book is strictly for informational and educational purposes.

Warning – Disclaimer

The purpose of this book is to educate and entertain. The author and/or publisher do not guarantee that anyone following these techniques, suggestions, tips, ideas, or strategies will become successful. The author and/or publisher shall have neither liability nor responsibility to anyone with respect to any loss or damage caused, or alleged to be caused, directly or indirectly by the information contained in this book.

ISBN: 098519460X
ISBN-13: 978-0-9851946-0-4

This book is dedicated to the loving memory of

Charles Francis McCormick
(9/3/1906 – 10/13/1976)
&
Catherine Mae (Bulock) McCormick
(4/2/1910 – 8/30/1985)

For the
dedication and diligence
love and devotion
care and concern
morals and ethics
understanding and compassion
faith
forgiveness
healing
integrity
persistence
goodness
kindness
and happiness
with which you lived your lives
and for teaching these values and ideals to your four sons
by word, deed, and example in a beautiful and powerful way
thank you.

be at peace, all is well, angels are near

Contents

Contents (continued)

Acknowledgements

I would like to acknowledge those people who graciously read the manuscript for this book before it was sent to the publisher. I thank them for finding typographical errors and for pointing out parts in the first draft that needed to be restated or made clearer. Thank you to my wife Rose, my daughters Tara Pienkowski, Erin Sloan, and Nicole Einhorn and to my dear friends Susan Jimerson and Sara Jimerson-Giglio. Without their reading over the rough draft and their good thoughts, this work would not have been brought to fruition. It was not only their proofreading, but also their reinforcement, support, and belief in the message that helped in ways that words cannot describe.

I sincerely thank Ralph Marston, motivational author of books and the Internet site http://greatday.com, "The Daily Motivator"© for very graciously giving his permission to use his quotes at the beginning of each section of the book. Ralph Marston is my mentor in life and I highly respect his work, his outlook on life, and his philosophy. You will read more about Ralph Marston in the introduction. Visit his website and be prepared to be inspired.

Thank you to my newspaper customers on my paper route when I was growing up—the people that you will read about in this book; thank you to the men and women who are a part of my rehabilitation groups and my grief groups and my hospital and church groups who teach me something every time we meet; thank you for teaching me the lessons of life.

Thank you to all who have crossed my path and continue to cross my path at the hospital where I am a chaplain, at the church where I am the parish deacon, and at the college where I teach and administer; thank you for the lessons of life you continue to teach me every day.

And, finally, thank you to my family for putting up with me.

Introduction

Life is like a _____. Go ahead, fill in the blank: Life is like a *what*? I recently asked that question to a group that I was conducting and each participant in the room got a chance to fill in the blank. Some used the familiar phrase of Forrest Gump, "Life is like box of chocolates; you never know what you're gunna get." Others used sentences like the following:

- Life is like a roller coaster filled with twists and turns and up and downs.
- Life is like a bunch of crayons; each day is a different color.
- Life is like a coloring book; sometimes I just want to color outside the lines.
- Life is like a fast moving train and I can't get off.
- Life is like a spinning top and I'm getting dizzier and dizzier.
- Life is like a symphony; each day plays out a beautiful song.

One of my favorites that one of my group members offered:

- Life is like good book; each day is a newly read page in the chapters of my life.

And I have a friend named Sara who reflects on life since the passing of her father in a very beautiful and profound way. She says:

- Life is like the ocean, sometimes it's rough while other times it's smooth; yet it is always beautiful, deep and continuous.

Life is different things to different people at different times. To me life is like a classroom; each day offers a valuable lesson to be learned. I mention this analogy because that is precisely what this little book is about. In particular, this book is based upon a series of lessons that I learned during a particular period in my life when I was growing up in a small town in upstate New York. These are lessons that I have learned and from which I have garnered a set of rules by which to live life in a peaceful, serene, and somewhat content and joyful way.

These rules were engraved in my mind from experiences as a young boy about ten or eleven years old. Each rule is based upon a true story of my own personal encounter with someone I met while I was a paperboy delivering my newspapers on my regular route; someone who taught me a valuable lesson about life experiences, how to live life.

As I look back at this period of time in my life, it was a period when I was carefree and somewhat naive about the realities of life. Life seemed less complicated as I went about my after-school chore every afternoon: folding my newspapers and placing them into my newspaper carrier bags, balancing them precariously on the handlebars of my bicycle, and then setting out to deliver the newspapers to my 120-plus customers for the next hour or so. From about 3:30 to 5:00 every weekday afternoon I would conscientiously deliver my newspapers to my customers, seemingly without a care in the world, diligently undertaking my responsibilities while at the same time absorbing a wealth of knowledge that I would apply throughout my life.

It was on Saturday mornings after delivering the "Early Bird Edition" from around 6:00 to 7:30 a.m., and after having a hearty breakfast prepared by my mom, that I would then set out to visit the customers on my paper route to do my weekly collection. At that time, back in the early 1960's the customer paid 7 cents per issue, six days a week; so I would collect 42 cents from those who paid on a weekly basis. If I collected from 100 customers, I would have a total $42.00 not counting generous tips some customers would give to me. Then that afternoon I would go to the office of *The Evening Tribune* to pay my weekly bill which might be around $38.00 leaving me a very good profit of almost $4.00 for the week—quite a substantial amount of money at that time.

And it was during those Saturday morning visits to my customers when I collected my weekly receipts for the newspaper that I also encountered the people that I write about in this book. People like Mrs. Stewart who was an elderly widow and for whom I was probably her only visitor for the entire week; Mr. Hart who suddenly stopped greeting me on Saturday's because he died unexpectedly (my first experience with death); Mr. and Mrs. Watson who showed me about the power of passion; David who taught me some characteristics that I chose not to aspire to, and so on. I have changed the names of some of the people, but the stories are real stories of true encounters.

Young and old, male and female, rich and poor, hard workers and slackers, honest people and those who were less than trustworthy; each one taught me something about life, something that has proven to be invaluable and worth much more than the $4.00 weekly profit I would spend on candy bars or movies and snacks.

Now that I am much older and wiser and as I look back at the people I met on my paper route and the lessons they taught me, I have come to the realization that what I learned can be summarized into these basic rules that make up what I call a manual for living a happy and content life, or a "how to" booklet on finding peace and contentment in a world that seems to be filled with stress and chaos.

The rules are not complicated or complex and are not meant to be difficult to follow in life but rather they are meant to be easy to follow rules. After all, life is meant to be enjoyed; we are supposed to be happy and have inner peace. Happiness and peace and joy are not meant to be complicated. We tend to make life complex by our worries, anxieties, misdirection, and misconceptions. Peace, joy, contentment and happiness are meant to be a part of our daily living experiences in a very beautiful and profound way. Life should be good and we should experience the rich blessings that unfold for us every day of our lives. We should be able to ground our lives in serenity and calmness every moment, and it is the goal of this book to help accomplish that.

✓ If you are searching for happiness and joy in your life…
✓ If your life is lacking peace and tranquility…
✓ If your life is void of meaning and there is something missing in your daily routine….
✓ If you question your purpose and wonder what life is all about…
✓ If you are lost and find your days without any kind of fulfillment…
✓ If you find that there is an emptiness that cannot be filled with money, friends, social outlets or other sources that you have attempted to use or abuse…
✓ If you are finding it more difficult to cope with the challenges of life or with stressful situations that seem to be occurring more frequently…

…then this little book containing some essential rules for happiness is meant for you.

I call it a manual, you may call it a learner's guide or a handbook or simply a booklet. The format is as follows for each of the nine rules:

    a. An inspirational quote from Ralph Marston (see below)
    b. A story from my paper route encounters that teach a lesson about the rule
    c. The Rule that applies to the lesson
    d. Some exercises on how to apply The Rule in your life
    e. A self quiz to determine your particular level or quotient relating to each rule

It is the goal of this book to have you learn how to apply these nine rules in your life so that you may ultimately experience profound peace, jubilant joy, heartfelt happiness, and continual contentment and in doing so to come to the realization that life is good and all is well.

And so, let me add one more "Gumperism" here: Life is like a manual, it is better to follow the instructions or else you get lost. Use the nine different rules that are presented here as a guide to finding that true happiness, true inner peace, true joy, and true contentment that you so intently desire in your life. Embrace life and enjoy it and savor the splendor of true and *unconditional* happiness.

One final note, I mentioned in the paragraph above that I use an inspirational quote from Ralph Marston. I consider Ralph Marston a modern day philosopher and great motivational writer, speaker, and thinker. Ralph Marston has an inspirational web site: http://greatday.com that offers a daily thought for the day that is always filled with positive affirmations that have to do with life, life experiences, and the trials and tribulations of everyday life. His thoughts are thoughts that I consider to be universal and touch the hearts and souls of every man, woman, and child in every culture and in every civilization; they are indeed profound.

His web page is entitled *The Daily Motivator* © and I would urge you to visit his site and join his many followers who listen to his powerful message every day. I consider Mr. Marston my mentor in life and quote him many times in the groups I conduct and in sermons and homilies that I give in the churches where I preach. Ralph Marston has graciously granted me permission to use his quotes in this book and for that I am forever grateful.

I end this *Introduction* and begin the *Manual* with a quote from Ralph Marston's *The Daily Motivator©* archives http://greatday.com

Silent Reflection

"For just a while, calm your thoughts. In this moment, simply be. There is much in your life, and there is much more to come. Yet you have always been, and you always are, more than enough. For a moment, let go of the way you appear and the things you've done. Feel the truth and power of who you are. In silence, there is much you can know. Beyond thought, there is much you can understand. Touch the person who always lives inside the person you are. Be immersed in the beauty and wonder of being. Feel the strength that is always there. And know that whatever may come, all is well."

~Ralph Marston, 'Silent Reflection,' The Daily Motivator©, December 24, 2008 http://greatday.com

Simplicity

"To gain an aptitude for simplicity, we must experience life directly. We must look not for complex hidden meanings, but rather for what is really there. We must accept on faith what our senses and sensibilities tell us. We must shut out the noise of anger, envy, regret, worry and deception, to experience the quiet power of simplicity."

~Ralph Marston, 'Simple Power,' The Daily Motivator ©, September 5, 1997 http://greatday.com

Mrs. Joseph and the Story of Simplicity

One of my first customers on my paper route was a family that lived on what was then State Street. They lived in a rickety old house that had open windows and open doors in the summer time so that you could see right through the house from one end to the other. There was very little inside: a torn old couch; a coffee table filled with dirty pots and pans that were overflowing from the kitchen; a kitchen stove that had not been cleaned in years and an even messier refrigerator. And instead of bedrooms with nicely decorated wallpaper and dressers and stands there were rooms with no doors that had cots with clothes scattered in bins that were stacked on top of one another.

The family was made up of the mother, Mrs. Joseph, and her four children of various ages, ranging from about one-year old to about six years old. I never saw Mr. Joseph, if there was a Mr. Joseph; either he was always working, or he was not a part of the picture at that time.

There was no car, no phone, no huge entertainment center, no extravagant window dressings, no closets filled with a selection of clothes or shoes to pick from, nothing extra, just the plain basic necessities of life. But week after week I could see that they had a roof over their heads, they had food on the kitchen table, they gathered together at mealtime and shared stories, and they had a home.

I remember distinctly on my Saturday visits how very warm and friendly Mrs. Joseph was when I came to collect my coins for the paper. I always felt bad about having to collect money, but she always greeted me with a big smile. She would retrieve her small change purse from her apron pocket and carefully open it up, spill out the few coins that were inside the purse and carefully and methodically count out exactly 42 cents. And with a big sigh and even bigger smile, she would always say, "There you are young man, keep deliver'n them papers 'cuz I sure do like to read'n my paper." Then we would talk for about five or ten minutes. I never left a customer without talking with them for a while.

She would tell me about how the littlest one was learning to walk or how the oldest one was doing in kindergarten. She would show me some of the "masterpieces" that the kids had colored with their crayons and were now hanging like paintings in an art gallery on the kitchen refrigerator. I could see the expression of love in her eyes and hear it in her voice. And I would always complement her and thank her and tell her what a wonderful family she had. And the next week when I would come to collect again, she would repeat the ritual all over again.

It was a wonderful learning experience for me because I learned that not everybody in life has a lot and that it does not take a lot of things to be happy. That was an important lesson for a young boy of ten or eleven years old to come to realize; and I must admit, that it took some years before it finally sank in.

Looking back at the Joseph family, what I learned was that in the midst of this household, that what they lacked in material things, they made up for in love.

And what I found out in the ensuing years was that this lesson I learned from the Joseph's can be applied to almost every aspect of life. One of the main ingredients to life is simplicity. Simplicity refers not just to the material possessions of life, but to the physical, emotional, and spiritual attributes of our minds, hearts, and souls.

The Rule of Simplicity

Consciously eliminate regrets, frustrations, failures, and guilt of the past. Do not add anxious worrisome thoughts about what may or may not happen tomorrow. As best you can, concentrate on the moment you are in and fulfill that moment with good thoughts and positive affirmations. Weigh in your mind the things you need as opposed to the things that you want in every aspect of your life. And realize that to downsize is to utilize the best of what you already have.

Simplicity involves four parts. First, consciously eliminate the regrets, frustrations, failures, and guilt of the past. For some, this may be more difficult than letting go of physical objects of our lives; but this is one of the most important parts of the rule. Some people try to get through life by thinking that they can be happy without eliminating regrets or guilt from the past. They "fake" their happiness and put on a wonderful façade, but in reality, they are only fooling themselves.

No matter how big of a smile they may put on, they are still hurting on the inside. You cannot substitute this important part of the rule with anything but the truth because to do so means that you are not being honest with yourself. When you try to cover up or hide the regrets, failures, or guilt of the past without dealing with it, you will ultimately pay the price. True happiness will never be found.

This step involves forgiveness, not just of others, but forgiveness of you. It may be helpful in completing this part by making a list of your failures or regrets or things you are frustrated about and consciously checking this list off as you play out in your mind past scenarios, knowing and realizing and coming to the understanding that you did the best you could and that there is nothing more that you can do. Forgiveness is a great healer, and healing begins with you.

The second section of the Rule of Simplicity reminds us not to add any anxious or worrisome thoughts about things that might or might not happen tomorrow. Worry is one of the most powerful and deadly self-defeating weapons that one can use against oneself. It stifles every aspect of your thinking and growth and virtually eliminates any positive spin we try to place on life. Agonizing, fretting, and being overly anxious and concerned are not healthy attributes to follow when trying to live a life of peace, joy and happiness.

The first two measures of the Rule of Simplicity lead to the third consideration which is to live for the moment; and not just *for* the moment but live *in* the moment. To live in the moment is to enjoy the peace and tranquility of who you are, where you are, what you are, and with what you have, right now, without adding or deleting anything. What a wonderful gift it is to be able to appreciate the moments of our lives and to savor those moments with the power of simplicity.

And finally, the last section of The Rule of Simplicity is a reminder to look at the things you need as opposed to the things you want and to realize that to downsize is to utilize the best of what you already have to its fullest potential. This "need versus want" philosophy may require a change in attitude and a complete restructuring of your personal philosophy of how you acquire things in life.   There is a Greek word for this changing of your attitude or outlook on life, it's called *Metanoia,* which literally means to breakdown and rebuild through a healing process. Your philosophy about how you acquire things may require you to experience a metanoia in every sense of its meaning.

There is a very popular phrase that is used quite a bit on television these days that denotes the philosophy of today's cultures: "Go big or go home." I never liked that phrase, probably because I always liked my home and I never had any problem in "going home" to begin with. I might change that phrase to reflect a more simple philosophy, one that embraces the Rule of Simplicity in my life. Rather than saying, "Go big or go home," I might say "Keep it simple, stay at home, and be happy."

Exercises in Simplicity

Exercise A

In applying simplicity in your own life, begin by asking yourself the following questions:

1. Do I have any unresolved regrets from the past that I can list as holding me down or holding me back?
2. Do I have anything that I feel guilty about from the past?
3. Have I failed at anything in the past and felt bad about that failure?

If you have answered yes to any of these questions, list the regrets or reasons for your guilt or failures; write a paragraph or two about why you feel the way you do, explain what happened and all that you have done to resolve the situation. Be at peace with what you have done. Then put it aside and out of your mind and out of your life once and for all.

Have you been able to forgive yourself totally and unconditionally for any and all things that have caused resentment, guilty or feelings of failure in the past? If not write yourself a "letter of forgiveness" beginning with Dear (your name): I forgive you completely for (list all the things you need to forgive yourself for). Go into great detail and list everything and anything that you need to be forgiven for. When you are done, sign the letter and then place the letter in envelope, seal it, address it to yourself and place a stamp on it and mail it to yourself if possible. If not, you can simply place the letter in a safe place and pull it out every so often whenever you need to be reminded of the fact that you have been forgiven. Once you have been totally and unconditionally forgiven, feel free to destroy the letter.

Exercise B

Do you find yourself worrying about things? Do you consider
yourself someone who worries needlessly about things that never
happen? Some form of worrying is healthy as it keeps us on our toes
and prepares us for situations; however over-worrying or anxiety
causes undue stress. Some people suffer from General Anxiety
Disorder which is to systematically worry about things, events, people,
and happenings so as to literally debilitate a person's life. This type of
worry is unhealthy and may require professional counseling.
However, here is an outline of things that you might do in order to
help combat the sensation of over-worrying in order to simplify your
life.

First, try to isolate the things that you are worrying about and untangle
those worrisome threads like strings of spaghetti and deal with each
strand one at a time. If you are worrying about the weather the next
day, what to wear, your son's activities, your finances, your
relationships; whatever the source, write it down, make a list, untangle
the many strands that make up the source of your worries.

Once your list is made, deal with each one head-on. Know that some
of the things you are worrying about cannot be changed, but must be
accepted. Have faith in yourself, have faith in others, have faith in
your source of Goodness, your God or your Higher Power. Do the
best you can with what you have and remember the adage that applies
to almost all situations: "This too shall pass." And one more adage I
like to add. Be at peace, all is well.

Deal with your list, put it in the proper context of reality, do the best
you can with what you have, accept what you must, trust and have
faith, realize that this too will pass, and that all will be well.

Exercise C

This exercise is simply to remember to stop and rest and realize that you don't have to rush every minute of the day. In the midst of your daily chores, tasks, duties, errands, responsibilities, jobs, and every day events and circumstances, STOP! Take a deep breath. Realize that life is beautiful and simple and meant to be enjoyed. In that moment, breathe in the splendor of surrendering to sweet serenity and surround yourself with the sounds of simplicity. Let this happen as long as you can and as many times as you can, safely and carefully, whenever possible.

Exercise D

Begin now to downsize with the material possessions in your life. Although this is something that you may think is for the elderly or those who are completing their journey of life; it is something to consider for the very young. Consider the philosophy "What do you need versus what do you want." Do you want to have three television sets, one for each room in the house, or do you only need one? Do you want to have 24 pairs of shoes or do you need... well, you get the picture. The best you can, try to downsize, keeping in mind that you still have to enjoy life. Downsize by utilizing what you have to fullest potential.

Finally, complete the Simplicity Quiz below to determine your own Simplicity Score. Place your score below and keep it in the back of your mind for later use.

The Simplicity Quiz

Answer the following questions and rate yourself according to the corresponding graphs to the best of your ability:

1. On a scale of 0-3 how do you rate your ability to deal with regrets of the past? Check a number box, 0 being regrets are a debilitating factor in your life and 3 being you have been able to get beyond regrets in your life and move on:

0	1	2	3
many regrets → a lot of regrets → some regrets → no regrets			

2. On a scale of 0-3 how do you rate your ability to deal with any guilt of the past? Check a number box, 0 being the fact that you still harbor guilt in your life and 3 being the fact that you have been able to get beyond guilt and move on:

0	1	2	3
much guilt → some guilt → guilt→ no guilt			

3. On a scale of 0-3 how do you rate your ability to forgive yourself for any events of the past? Check a number box, 0 being you have not been able to forgive yourself and 3 being you have forgiven yourself completely and you are able to move on:

0	1	2	3
not able to forgive → forgive little → forgive some → completely forgive			

4. On a scale of 0-3 how do you rate your *worry quotient*? Check a number box, 0 being very low and you worry about everything and 3 being very good, you don't worry about anything and you are able to deal with life as it comes along:

0	1	2	3
worry about → everything	worry about → most things	worry bout → some things	do not worry at all

5. On a scale of 0-3 how do you rate your ability to live in the moment, that is forget things of the past and not think about the future. Are you able to stop and enjoy life without rushing through it? Check a number box, 0 if you are not able to enjoy the moment and 3 if you can live for the moment and "stop and smell the roses":

0	1	2	3
I cannot live → in the moment at all	I can live in → the moment sometimes	I can live in → the moment most times	I can live in the moment at all times

6. On a scale of 0-3 how do you rate your ability to downsize your lifestyle? Have you been able to get rid of excess materialistic possessions and utilize what you have to its fullest? Do you follow the maxim "need versus want" in your life? Check a number box, 0 being the fact that you have not been able to downsize at all and 3 being the fact that you have downsized considerably:

0	1	2	3
I have not been → able to downsize at all	I have been → able to down-size very little	I have been → able to down-size some	I have been able to down-size a lot

Now add together your scores from the six questions above and write your total score here:

My Simplicity Score _____

Keep your score handy as it will be used in a final calculation to determine your total Happiness Quotient at the end of the book. For now, let's see how you rate in terms of applying simplicity in your life.

If your Simplicity Score is between 14 – 18 you are probably following the Rule of Simplicity very well in your life and that is a good thing because you will find the other rules for happiness will fall into place a little bit easier

If your Simplicity Score is between 9 – 13 you are following the Rule of Simplicity somewhat in your life. You may want to check those areas in your life where you can improve a little bit as they apply to the specific applications of the rule.

If your Simplicity Score is between 4 – 8 you may want to take a look at where you can specifically improve your simplicity quotient by following some of the exercises in the book that pertain to those areas where you are weak.

If your Simplicity Score is between 0 – 3 you may want to complete the exercises again, re-evaluate your lifestyle, and then retake the

Simplicity Quiz to see if you can improve your application of the Rule of Simplicity in your life.

Keep in mind that there is no scientific or psychological basis for the testing material contained herein but the material is for educational purposes only and the main goal of this book, as stated previously, is for you to achieve happiness in your life.

Finally, review The Rule of Simplicity, the exercises, your scores, and then evaluate yourself in relation to where you want to be. Learn and practice the Rule of Simplicity as often as you can in your daily life. The more you become conscious of it, the more you apply it, the more you practice it, the happier you will be.

Humility

"Do not make the mistake of discarding your humility...for humility keeps you reasonable, respectful, thankful, thoughtful and realistic, and those are all qualities essential for continued success. Humility reminds you that in order to receive value, you must create value in equal measure. While it is certainly possible to accomplish things without humility, those accomplishments will be empty and short-lived. Those people who enjoy meaningful success and fulfillment year after year and decade after decade are those people who know the value of humility."

~Ralph Marston, 'Humility,' The Daily Motivator ©, October 13, 2007
http://greatday.com

Dr. Eddy and Mr. & Mrs. Lent and a Story about Humility

This is the story of three people on my paper route, a man and a couple whom I would occasionally meet when they would happen to be outside at their homes when I was delivering the newspaper, or they would be at home on Saturday morning when I did my weekly collecting.

The first is the story of Dr. Theodore Eddy who lived in a huge, wonderfully built house on Seneca Street. Dr. Eddy was a local doctor and went to no expense at making his house one of the most attractive in the small city where I grew up. And being the young impressionable boy that I was, I considered his house to be a mansion. It was probably a very modest house by some standards, but to me it was a castle. It had stained glass windows; a driveway that you could turn around in; six huge white pillars on the front porch; an archway where guests could be left off before entering the house; a six-car garage filled with two Cadillac's, a Lincoln Continental, and two or three antique cars that were in pristine condition; and it was adorned in the most ornate inlaid brick design that I had ever seen.

To say the least, Dr. Eddy was well off, and he let it be known that he could afford most anything he wanted. But what I remember most about Dr. Eddy was his character and his temperament. In particular, on one occasion when I delivered the newspaper after 5:00 p.m. in the evening, he made it a point to telephone the offices of *the Evening Tribune* and not only complain about the poor quality of service he was receiving from his paperboy (me), but also that he, Dr. Eddy, was not used to being treated with such disrespect. I became aware of his complaint from a telephone call from the circulation manager that evening. The manager was totally sympathetic to my plight and realized that it was not my fault.

On another occasion when I inadvertently rang his doorbell on a Saturday morning informing him that I was collecting my weekly fee for the newspaper, he immediately went into a fuming frenzy about how it was beneath him to pay a few cents each week and that he paid his bill by the year at the main office. After having the door slammed in my face, I left the house feeling about as tiny as an ant in the bottom of the Grand Canyon.

Dr. Eddy was not a very humble man, and from what I learned later in life, was not very well respected among his fellow citizens, community members, or even his family.

A few houses down from Dr. Eddy on the same side of the street there was another house that was very modestly built but attractive. It was occupied by a man and his wife and their son who owned a local clothing store. Mr. and Mrs. Lent were extremely well off and could probably afford anything they wanted; and yet they never appeared to live beyond their means.

There was something very humbling about the Lent's, Mr. Lent was always doing his own lawn work, Mrs. Lent did her own shopping, their son played sports and they went to all his games, they donated to local charities, and when you went into their Main Street clothing store, you were always greeted with a warm smile and an appreciative conversational tone that you could tell was genuine.

On my weekly visits to the Lent household, Mrs. Lent would answer the door, but Mr. Lent would always make it a point to get up from his large over-stuffed den chair where he had been smoking his vanilla-flavored aromatic pipe and greet me with a hand shake, a smile, and the inevitable question, "How are you doing this morning, Bob?" He would then reach in his pocket, pull out a fifty-cent piece, flip it in the air to me and add, "Keep the change, and thanks for putting the paper on the porch." Wow, did that make me feel good. Not just the fact

21

that he had given me an eight-cent tip, but more importantly, the recognition that I had done a good job and he noticed it. Leaving the Lent household was much different than leaving the Eddy home.

Of the people mentioned above, who do you think was happier: Dr. Eddy or the Lent's? Who do you think practiced the virtue of humility, and in doing so, showed their true strength and character? Of course, it was Mr. and Mrs. Lent who, in my eyes, were people whom I epitomized and people whom I wanted to pattern my life after when I grew up.

The lesson I learned from Dr. Eddy was simple but lasting: rude, inconsiderate, snobbish, and selfish people are very often trying to boost their own ego and are not respected. On the other hand, what I learned from the Lent's was just the opposite: humility builds strength and character which in turn breeds fulfillment, success, and happiness.

The Rule of Humility

When in the course of daily events you have any opportunity to learn from someone, grasp that moment with full abandon and savor those times like treasures more valuable than gold. Never underestimate the power of humility for in humbleness you will earn the respect of every person your path of life encounters. Humility is the secret to inner acceptance which leads to great peace of mind, and peace of mind leads to happiness.

One of the greatest attributes of the monks in ancient times was their humble mindedness, their ability to remain at peace with themselves in spite of the conflicts and chaos of the world around them. This is true of even the most modern day monasteries and the rule of order that the monks follow. There is an abbey near where I live called the Abbey of the Genesee and I visit it quite often in order to find peace, solitude and calmness. It is a very serene place where the monks follow rules of life that bring them closer to God. In their humbleness they find peace, solitude, and happiness.

True inner peace and happiness that is lasting comes from a self-confidence that is grounded in courage and strength and manifests itself with words and actions that are effective yet gentle. One of the qualities of highly effective people is humility, humility tempered with wisdom. And when humility and wisdom are used hand-in-hand, it leads to happiness and peace. Humility leads to an inner awareness and confidence that transcends egotism and self-righteousness but unfolds in the splendor of blissfully being.

A member of one of the groups that I was conducting recently told the story of how he had turned his life completely around from being an arrogant, egotistical, rude, and obnoxious person to following a life of humility and how he was much happier since he had done so. When I asked him how he was able to do that, how he was able to change from arrogant to humble mindedness he said it took practice.

Like most good things in this world that we wish to acquire, if it doesn't come naturally, it takes practice. If humility does not come easy for you, practice the virtue, adopt it as a conscientious outlook on life, and it will get easier and easier to adopt as a rule of life and a key to happiness.

Exercises in Humility

Humility often involves emptying our self of our pride and egotism and allowing others to help us, teach, or offer advice. For some, this is a very difficult thing to do in life because we consider ourselves mature, wise or experts in our field. To humble one's self is to be open to other opinions and to void ourselves of any preconceived judgmental assumptions that we may have regarding people, places, or events.

Exercise A

Find a topic or subject that you are not familiar with and ask someone who has knowledge in that area to help you to understand the material a little better. This could be something that you always wanted to know about, for example: music, horses, the Internet, Facebook, etc. Admit that you don't know much about the subject, seek out someone who does, and ask them to help you learn the subject.

Exercise B

 Ask someone to evaluate something that you do and then have them give their opinion on how you can improve; have them not only give you healthy criticism, but also their advice. Of course, who you choose to evaluate your performance should have some knowledge about what you are having them criticize. For example, you may want to have your mother-in-law evaluate your cooking and taste the food you have prepared and give you some advice on how to better prepare a meal (maybe not!). If you are a teacher, have a fellow teacher watch your class and see if he can give you some advice. If you are a bowler, ask other bowlers for tips on how to bowl better and so on.

Exercise C

Find something that someone did a nice job on and give them a congratulatory compliment; not a false one that appears to be concocted and just made up out of pity, but a real, genuine compliment for a really fine job that was well done. Do this more than once, in fact, do it as many times as you possibly can and continue to do it.

Exercise D

Think of a recent experience where you learned something from someone by watching them or by listening to them or by merely being with them. Write this down on a piece of paper and then take just a moment to reflect on what you learned. This does not have to be a grand experience, but it can be something as simple as a new way to get a lid of a jar that is too tight or how to remove dried wax stains from a carpet or clothing. Thank that person for what you learned.

The Humility Quiz

In the following quiz, give yourself +0 points for each no answer and +1 point for each yes answer. Total your score at the end and record it in the space marked My Humility Score. Keep your score handy as it will be used at the end of the book. Answer the questions as they relate to your experiences BEFORE you completed the exercises above.

In the last two weeks before completing the Humility Exercises, have you:	No +0	Yes +1
Admitted that you did not know something?		
Admitted that you were wrong at anytime?		
Complimented someone for a job well done?		
Asked someone for help?		
Accepted criticism or the opinion of another?		
Learned something from someone?		
Remember, do not count the exercises you completed above.		

Now add together your scores from the six questions above and write your total score here:

My Humility Score _____

Keep this score along with your other scores as they will be used in a final calculation to determine your total Happiness Quotient at the end of the book. For now, let's see how you rate in terms of applying humility in your life.

If you scored:	You may:
5-6	have great humility
3-4	be somewhat humble
1-2	be somewhat vain
0	probably be conceited

Finally, no matter what your score, try to practice humility in your life endeavors and you will find that you will be a happier person and those around you will be happier as well.

Acceptance

"It is through total acceptance of what is that you gain total control of what can be. By allowing life to come to you, you empower your purpose to radiate out from you. You cannot successfully fight against what is. For the moment you choose to fight, you're fighting against a past that cannot be changed. Live from a place of deep-seated peace. Instead of jumping into a reaction at every turn of events, exude a consistent, confident purpose. Lovingly accept every bit of life as it comes your way. And you will always find much to truly love."

~Ralph Marston, 'Total Acceptance,' The Daily Motivator ©, August 9, 2010 http://greatday.com

"Take a deep breath. Relax. Accept the person you are. Accept the people and the world around you. Bring peace, patience, learning and accomplishment to your life by practicing acceptance."

~Ralph Marston, 'Acceptance,' The Daily Motivator ©, August 10, 1996 http://greatday.com

The Story of Billy and the Lesson of Acceptance

One of the side streets that I delivered papers on contained houses that were very close together and what might be considered in somewhat poorer condition as compared to other sections of the city. It was a very small, one-way street with worn out houses and worn out people. At one end of the street, on the corner, was a large white tenement house where nothing but old people lived. It was run by an old lady named Mrs. Bradley who lived downstairs. There were creaky steps that led upstairs where it was always dark because the windows were covered over with big dirty drapes that looked like they had never been cleaned. And it was smelly; it smelled like a combination of tobacco smoke and the stench of urine that had not been cleaned from bedding.

I never looked forward to going upstairs to collect from the one or two tenants who may have taken the newspaper for a short time. I didn't like it because it scared me.

At the other end of the street was a large brick house with a family that always had children running around in diapers and dogs and cats all over the property, leaving their messes that were never cleaned up.

In between these two houses at either end of the street there was a collection of various households that contained a variety of men, women, and children. Preston Avenue turned out to be one of the most influential classrooms in terms of learning experiences. I learned more from the customers on this little street than I did in some of the college classes that I have taken in my lifetime. I learned about the reality of life and I learned how to apply what I learned into these rules of life. I learned a great deal from this tiny little street called Preston Avenue.

One of the most meaningful rules I acquired about life came from a valuable lesson I learned from a little boy who lived on this street. The little boy's name was Billy and the lesson I learned was acceptance.

Billy lived in a large brown house in the center of Preston Avenue; it was a dark brown, shabby looking house that needed painting. It needed windows and a new roof, the doors weren't level so they never shut tight, the porch was ready to fall down, and there were a few steps leading up to the porch that were missing.

Billy was seven or eight years old, he had blonde hair, he was very skinny, and there was something unusual that I noticed about Billy when I first met him and his mother, Billy never walked. Whenever I was at the house I saw that his mom would always carry him from place to place or he would always be sitting down.

One Saturday morning when I was collecting, I noticed that Billy had big, dark brown braces on both legs. I didn't know whether this prevented him from walking or whether they were used to help him stand up or what they were for. I also noticed that he had two metal hand crutches over in the corner. This was my first encounter with someone who had a handicap or disability, someone who was not able to do things that I could do and was challenged by things that I might take for granted.

I distinctly remember asking myself if Billy ever thought about not being able to play baseball or run down the street; not being able play sports in school or do the other things that young children at his age do. And I remember seeing the care and compassion that his mother displayed when she picked him up and moved him from his chair to the table or from the house to the porch and how she would make sure that he had the things he needed.

This encounter with Billy, and later encounters in my life with other people who were similarly challenged, led to a very valuable lesson that I learned. That lesson was to accept who and what I am and to do the best I can with what I have. To realize that there are some things in life that cannot be changed and that to fight against them is useless. To make positive choices in life and to optimistically look forward to each new day with hope and determination that is filled with the power of acceptance.

A life without acceptance is like a life that is doomed for unhappiness. If one cannot accept the realities of life and be able to deal with them in a healthy and positive way, then discontentment and disharmony are the predictable outcomes for such a person.

Billy had a physical challenge that he accepted in his life, and he did that very well. He was always smiling and cheerful and I don't ever remember him complaining. There were times when he would be gone for periods of weeks, times when I later learned that he was confined to the hospital for complications. But then he would always return home, smiling and cheerful, greeting each day with acceptance.

The Rule of Acceptance

There are events and circumstances in life that cannot be changed or altered because they are out of our control. Acceptance of this fact of life relieves the mind and frees the spirit to accomplish great tasks and to ground our lives with an inner peace beyond description. The acceptance of who we are leads to an awareness of what we can do which in turn creates a euphoric sensation in our lives that generates a genuine and lasting purpose in life. Acceptance is a major component to happiness, satisfaction, peace, and joy in all of life's endeavors.

Acceptance of circumstances and events in life that cannot be changed must be total and unconditional. Acceptance of who we are with all of our faults and failures as well as our good points cannot be something that is done half way. Acceptance of past events that cannot be altered, current events that are solidified in life's situations and future events that are beyond our control is necessary for a positive attitude toward ourselves and those around us.

This element of Acceptance is fundamental to the development of a healthy, successful, and happy attitude toward life itself. Acceptance does not mean that we have to cave in to all of the problems and frustrations of life or that we have to become slaves to every disappointing event in our lives. There are lots of things in life that we can change and should change. It is those things that we cannot change that we need to accept. The first stanza of the *Serenity Prayer* by Richard Niebuhr talks about acceptance in a very beautiful and meaningful way:

God grant me the serenity to ACCEPT the things I CANNOT change; the courage to change the things I can; and the wisdom to know the difference.

There is a little booklet published by Abbey Press called *Acceptance: the Way to Serenity and Peace of Mind*, which was first published in 1960. It was written by Vincent P. Collins who was also a Roman Catholic priest. I knew Fr. Collins when I was a young boy growing up, he was assigned to the church that I attended and where I was an alter server. He was a remarkable person who had a somewhat of a troubled life but wrote some brilliant books based upon his experiences in life.

His little booklet *Acceptance* is only 24 pages in length and yet the message contained in those pages has changed the lives of millions of people who have been touched by the simplicity of its message. It has sold millions of copies and is still published today, over fifty years later. Fr. Collins uses the Serenity Prayer on the last page. His message is based on one word "acceptance."

You can gain happiness, peace, contentment, fulfillment, and joy by following acceptance in your daily living experiences. If you can temper what you say and what you do every day with Acceptance you will be healthier and happier.

Exercises in Acceptance

Another word for acceptance is tolerance, are you tolerant of people and situations in your life? Sometimes tolerance involves patience. Try some of the following exercises to become more acceptable, more tolerant, and more patient.

Exercise A

The next time you are in the supermarket or mall and you have completed your purchases, rather than looking for the shortest line, look for the longest line. Accept the fact that you may have to wait an extra few minutes to leave the store. In fact, if there is someone behind you, invite them to go ahead of you to make your length of time even longer. Accept the fact that you may not be out of the store as quickly as you may have wanted to be. Try to accept life as it comes with all of its challenges, difficulties, frustrations, and long lines at the supermarket or mall.

Exercise B

The next time you are asked by your spouse or friend or someone you are going out to dinner with where you want to go, tell them that the choice is completely their choice and that you will accept whatever they decide to do. Or let someone else decide the movie or play you are going to see. Accept the fact that you have turned complete control over to someone else in making a decision.

Exercise C

In driving home or driving to the store or driving on the freeway, rather than driving faster than the person next to you or trying to get to your destination in the shortest possible time; rather than trying to beat the light before it turns yellow or red; rather than half-stopping at each stop sign; drive the speed limit, stop completely at each stop sign, drive courteously, and accept the fact that you don't have to drive like a maniac to get to your destination. Try it!

Exercise D

Make a list of all of your strengths and all of your weaknesses. For each strength that you have, tell yourself how great you are and what a great job you are doing. For each weakness that you have, tell yourself how great you are and what a great job you are doing. Accept yourself for who and what you are and know that you are doing a wonderful job with what you have and you are doing the best you can.

The Acceptance Quiz

Check the box under the answer that best fits your response to the following questions about your attitude toward acceptance. Try to answer the questions without thinking too deeply into them; your first response should be your answer:

	None of the time +0	Some of the time +1	Most of the time +2	All of the time +3
Are you able to accept your faults?				
Do you accept others without trying to change them?				
Are you patient with others?				
Are you tolerant of others difficulties or plights?				
Can you accept defeat easily?				

Now add together your scores from the five questions above and write your total score here:

My Acceptance Score _____

Keep this score along with your other scores as they will be used in a final calculation to determine your total Happiness Quotient at the end of the book. For now, let's see how you rate in terms of applying acceptance in your life.

If your Acceptance Score was between 12 – 15 you are probably pretty well suited in terms of your acceptance of who you are and where you are going in life. That is a good thing. You are also probably pretty tolerant of those around you and are not judgmental.

If your score was between 8 – 11 you are somewhat acceptable of those around you and your own life. You may need to work on accepting your weaknesses and your faults and you also may need to practice acceptance and tolerance.

If your score was between 4 – 7 you may want to practice the virtue of acceptance in your life by trying the exercises and conscientiously applying the virtue of acceptance the best you can in your everyday affairs. This conscientious attitude may require a complete shift in your attitude of how you see yourself and others around you.

The same thing applies if your score was between 0 -3. In fact, you may want to consider enrolling in specialized courses that deal with how to become more accepting in your life or reading books on the virtue of acceptance.

Finally, in all instances, practice acceptance every chance you get. The more accepting you become, the closer you get to your ultimate goal of achieving unconditional happiness.

Deacon Robert W. McCormick

Integrity

"Integrity is something that a lot of people talk about, but to have integrity, it takes more than talk. It's easy to show integrity when things are going good. The real test of a person's integrity is how they perform under adversity. The winners in life realize that life is interconnected -- that the things you do today will come back to you at some point...so even when things are going bad, winners perform with integrity."

~Ralph Marston, The Daily Motivator©, 'Integrity,' March 15, 1996
http://greatday.com

"Anything that stands in the way of your integrity will eventually bring you down."

~Ralph Marston, 'A Continuing Drain,' The Daily Motivator©, April 26, 2000 http://greatday.com

The Integrity of David (or the lack thereof)

As I mentioned earlier, one of the best classrooms of my life was Preston Avenue. The people I met and events that happened on Preston Avenue when I was delivering the weekday newspapers or collecting on Saturday mornings resulted in what I refer to as "teaching moments" in my life. They weren't earth-shattering events by any means, but they were little things in life that later on, as I grew older and wiser and reflected back on those moments, offered me morals and values, principles and ethics, rules to live by that helped me appreciate the goodness of life and instill a genuine feeling of happiness, bliss, and peacefulness.

One of the most important lessons I learned at an early age was the lesson of honesty, fair play, candor, or integrity. I consider Integrity as a fundamental rule of life. I learned about integrity in a roundabout way through Mrs. Jackson.

Mrs. Jackson lived in the very first house on Preston Avenue. She lived in the upper apartment by herself. She was probably in her mid-60s or early 70s, but it was hard to tell because I only saw her once or twice when I was delivering the newspaper. As a rule, I would always leave the paper at the top of the stairs for her every day; and when I collected on Saturday, she would always, without any deviation from her routine, always do something that no other customer had ever done.

Inside the hallway that led to the steps going up to her apartment was a small wooden desk that greeted those who entered the house. On top of the desk there was a ceramic tomato about the size and color and shape of a real tomato. In fact, the tomato looked very real, but if you pulled on the stem, the top came off so that you could put items inside of the tomato.

Every week, without failure, Mrs. Jackson would leave exactly 42 cents in change inside of that tomato for me to collect for the newspaper. Every week without failure I would go up the stairs of the front porch, enter the front door into the hallway and go to the desk, carefully pick up the tomato and take the top off, and then cautiously pour out the change into my hand. I didn't count the money because I knew there was always 42 cents. It had become a habit, a ritual that I so enjoyed. I always looked for that tomato and always knew the money would be there waiting for me.

Then one Saturday morning, it was not there! As I lifted the top of the tomato and tipped it into my hand, nothing came out. I carefully examined the inside of the ceramic tomato, wondering if the coins had gotten stuck, I searched the floor thinking that I might have spilled the coinage accidentally, and I even looked inside the drawer of the desk, thinking there might be some change in there that she forgot to put into the tomato. Sometimes Mrs. Jackson would leave a small note for me, so I looked again to see if there was any note—nothing! I just could not believe my eyes! After two or three years of being conditioned to always collect my 42 cents by taking the lid of the ceramic tomato; I was awe struck and devastated and didn't know what to do.

Should I knock on the door and ask Mrs. Jackson for the money? Should I wait until next week to see if she would pay me twice the amount, which some customers often did? Or should I just ignore it and go on my way to the next customer. I chose the latter, hoping that Mrs. Jackson would come to her senses and realize that I needed my "tomato-fix," my mere 42 cents to satisfy my needs and make me happy once again. Dejected, I left the house and went on to my next customer.

As it turned out, it was during this time that I was asked by the circulation manager of *The Evening Tribune* if I would help train another carrier boy, show him how to deliver the papers and what to do when collecting from customers. I gladly offered my services, and for one week, a boy named David shadowed me on my route to learn the ropes, what the job of a newspaper carrier was all about.

I must say that I was not impressed with David's character, his work ethic, or his demeanor with customers. I found myself having to explain to David how to respect customers and how to treat them nicely. He had a lot to learn, and I don't think it ever sank in.

The Saturday before my traumatic tomato tragedy I had taken David around on my collection route and shown him how to politely collect the money from the customers and how to visit with them. I taught him that it was proper not to just collect the money and leave but to stay and talk a while. I showed him how to treat customers, which customers preferred to pay weekly and which ones paid by the month and so on. I also showed David where some of the customers left their money for me to collect, including Mrs. Jackson's tomato.

I was to meet David one last time to see if he had any final questions about how to deliver the newspapers or how to collect the receipts. It happened to be the day I didn't find any money in the tomato. I met Dave at Leo's Market, right around the corner from Preston Avenue. We got off our bicycles and entered the store and both went to the cooler to get a Fawn root beer and then he grabbed a bag of potato chips and I went for a bag of cheese corn. We walked up to the counter and were greeted by the cashier with a friendly smile. I paid my money for my snack and soda with a dollar bill and got my change back.

I watched as David reached into his pocket and pulled out a handful of change, it was exactly 42 cents. Seeing the exact change kind of peaked my suspicion but what really put the "lid on the tomato" was the note that fell out of his pocket. Every so often Mrs. Jackson would leave a little note, telling me that she appreciated my putting the newspaper at the top of the steps. It was always scribbled in pencil on a torn piece of notebook paper and always the same wording, "Thank you for putting the paper by my door." My heart sank when I saw the note fall on the floor and I picked it up and read it. I asked David where he got the note and he said something about his mother giving him the note as he ran out of the store leaving his Fawn root beer, chips, and an awe-struck eleven year-old boy.

I never saw David again, frankly, I didn't want to. That was my first encounter with someone who was consciously dishonest. I never met anyone who purposely had stolen anything or cheated and it was a new experience for me. It taught me a valuable lesson, one that, as time tempered my life I learned to apply to many other situations.   The world is filled with honest and dishonest people, and, unfortunately, you have to deal with both. How you deal with them sometimes a test of your own integrity.

The Rule of Integrity

On the journey of life you will meet many people. Some will be as honest as the day is long while others will take advantage of you and seek to connive and manipulate every aspect of your being. You must be on guard and discern in your heart those who are pure and those who have motives that are untrustworthy. Concerning your own self, integrity is the highest form of self respect and inner awareness that leads to true and lasting contentment, happiness and blissfulness. The adage, "To thine own self be true," means to live with integrity in your heart, your mind, your soul, your self, and every facet of your life. Integrity is more than a state of mind; it is a state of being, a state of existence, a state of daily accomplishment that manifests itself in word and in deed; what you say and what you do.

I once asked a group I was conducting what the word "integrity" meant to them. Most of them came up with some pretty standard definitions dealing with truth and honesty and being true to themselves.   And everyone agreed that one of the most fundamental aspects of integrity involved an element of self-awareness and an element of being conscious of the difference between right and wrong; and then going a step above that, being able to apply the rule of "right and wrong" in every situation, even when no one is looking.

And that element of applying the rule of "good and bad" to a situation when nobody was looking seemed to be a pretty good standard by which most of the members in my group measured integrity.

If you can do what you are supposed do, what is right, even when nobody is looking; if you can hold yourself accountable even when nobody else is going to be there to hold you accountable; if you can give it all you got—110 percent, even when no one is there to see what you are doing; then that is a pretty good measurement of someone who lives their life by the Rule of Integrity.

Integrity is more than a mind-set, it is a characteristic that highly effective leaders have chosen and adopted as a personal philosophy of life. They manifest in just about every aspect of their life from their work habits to their family life. They don't have to hide things or cover things up or make excuses but everything is out in the open and clear. You can tell a person with integrity because they are usually reliable, open, honorable, and have a good world view.

When you adopt integrity as a major characteristic in your lifestyle, you are adopting one of the most honored and treasured universal qualities of life that transcends generations and cultures from the beginning of time.

Anyone who lives a life without integrity is doomed to a life of false hope, misery, and temporary platitudes of pseudo-euphoric bliss. On the other hand, those who live their life with integrity find a true and lasting inner peace that manifests itself in completeness, contentment, joy, and happiness.

An Exercise in Integrity

Ponder the following scenarios and write a brief paragraph or think about how you would handle the following situations:

Scenario A

You are walking down the street, it is late at night and there is nobody around at all. You happen to see a bag on the side of the sidewalk just lying halfway in the grass almost hidden from view. As you get closer you see that it's a brown sack that's bulging. You approach the bag, pick it up, and very cautiously look inside. Inside the bag you see stacks and stacks of hundred dollar bills, all neatly bound with wrappers that say $1000 on them. There are at least 50 stacks of the $1000 wrapped bills. You close the bag, put it under your arm and walk home as quickly as you can.

Now think about or write a brief paragraph explaining what the next thing is that you would do with the bag of money.

Scenario B

You are at the grocery store and you pay the clerk for your groceries and she gives you back your change. When you get home you find that the clerk accidently gave you a $20 bill rather than a $1 bill so you have $19 more than you should.

Now think about or write a brief paragraph explaining what the next thing is that you would do with the extra $19 that you have.

Scenario C

You are at work and the boss has left town, there is no one else in the office and it is a beautiful sunny day outside. It is about 1 o'clock in the afternoon and you are supposed to work until 5 p.m. even though you don't have to punch in or out. Your boss just expects you to work from 9 – 5 every day. Imagine that you get a call from a friend who invites you to go to the beach or to an afternoon ballgame. There is no one else around; no one will know if you leave early or not.

Think about or write a brief paragraph explaining what you would do.

Scenario D

You and a friend took it upon yourselves to build a handicap access ramp for a neighbor. You both worked very hard in completing the job and you spent a lot of your own money for the material, at least

$500, and spent about a week building the ramp. When the job is done, the person you built the ramp for sent a thank you note to your friend and thanked him for the wonderful job he did in building the ramp and donating his time and money. You were never mentioned.

Think about or write a brief paragraph explaining what you would do.

The Integrity Quiz

Regarding the Exercise in Integrity and the four scenarios, answer the following questions by placing an X in the box that corresponds best to what you thought about or wrote in your paragraph.

	+0	+1	+2
In Scenario A above did you:	Keep the money	Try to find the owner	Turn the money over to the police
In Scenario B above did you :	Keep the extra change	Donate the change to charity	Return the change to the store
In Scenario C above did you:	Leave work immediately	Stay to get all your work done but left earlier than usual	Stay at work until 5 p.m.
In Scenario D above did you:	Tell the person who wrote the note that she forgot you	Tell your friend that you were upset	Let it pass without saying anything to anybody

Now total up your score and write it here:

My Integrity Score _____

Keep your score handy because it will be used to determine your total Happiness Score at the end of the book. For now, let's see what your total Integrity Quotient means.

Your Integrity Quotient meaning:	score
You are probably a very honest person with great integrity and honesty	7-8
You probably have pretty good standards most of the time	4-6
You may need to practice learning about integrity in your life	0-3

Finally, if you can become mindfully conscious of events and happenings in your life that revolve around truth, honesty, and integrity and try to conscientiously apply good, morally ethical principles, then integrity can be something you strive to achieve. I don't know whether it can be taught, but it can be observed in others and serve as an inspiration. It can be an example that you set for others. The more you apply integrity, the happier your life will be.

Deacon Robert W. McCormick

Persistence

"Even if the challenges are immense and the obstacles are many, step forward and live the life you choose to live. Even if you get knocked down again and again, get right back up and get going. With enough persistence, any goal is within your reach. Even if no one believes you, insist on being truthful. Each new day brings you more experience, wisdom and effectiveness. Even if you've been deeply disappointed in the past, focus on the positive possibilities".

~Ralph Marston, 'Even If,' The Daily Motivator©, January 6, 2012 http://greatday.com

"Persistence is not a complicated or inaccessible strategy. All you have to do is choose to keep going. Persist, and the small steps forward add together to create great advances. Persist, and even the setbacks will eventually work in your favor."

~Ralph Marston, 'With Persistence,' The Daily Motivator©, December 19, 2011 http://greatday.com

What Drives Persistence

One of the longest and busiest streets on my paper route was Seneca Street. This street contained a number of businesses including at least five gas stations, two auto car dealerships, and two fraternal organizations or social clubs. I could see the daily activities that occurred day in and day out in the businesses as the employees of the gas stations and auto dealerships went about their workday. I didn't know it at the time, but I began to observe a work ethic that was present in the men and women that came to work every day and the jobs that they did.

That was important for a young boy at my age to see, this persistence and perseverance with which they performed their work. I know it had a profound effect on me and made me work a little bit harder in doing my job as a paper boy. It also affected my personal view about work as I grew older and began working in part-time jobs while in college and then later as I undertook full-time jobs in my various careers and vocations as a teacher, school administrator, minister, writer, and chaplain.

This is a collective story, it's the story of Stan who worked at the Oldsmobile dealership, the men and women who worked at the Pontiac and Cadillac garage, George who worked at the Texaco gas station, Bill who worked at the Esso gas station, John who worked at the Gulf gas station, and Rodney who owned and operated his very own Rotary gas station, all of these men and women taught me a very valuable lesson about discipline, perseverance, and persistence in life and how important it is to follow a basic rule of persistence in living a happy life.

Stan would greet me every day at the garage door in the back of the Oldsmobile dealership; he was one of the mechanics who worked on the cars and trucks. He would be covered with grease from head to foot; there was not a clean spot on his Khaki uniform or his hands or face. He would be waiting for me every day with a smile and a snide remark about the paper not being worth the money he paid for it. But he would always be there every day, rain or shine, snow or sleet, he would be at work. There was something about his persistence that I looked up to and admired.

One afternoon when I got there a little bit earlier than usual, I walked over to where he was working on a car and I noticed his tool chest where he kept all his tools. There, taped above an oily rag and a greasy vice grip was a picture of his family, his wife and two small children. Looking at the picture of his family made me appreciate why he did what he did. It made me understand a little better why he came to work every day and got greasy and messy and worked from 6 in the morning until sometimes 4 or 5 in the afternoon, it was for his family. His persistence was grounded in love.

I saw the same drive, ambition, and perseverance in George who was in his 80s and his son Dick who was in his 50s, they both worked at a Texaco gas station on Seneca Street. The son would take care of his dad and make sure that he was okay, even though he couldn't do what he used to do when he was younger. I saw it present in Rodney who had a very special reason for persevering because his wife and baby lived above the gas station that he owned on Seneca Street. I remember the day he opened his Rotary gas station and his family moving in upstairs. I remember watching him hammer the sign above the front door of the gas station that read *"George Statton, Proprietor,"* and the pride and joy that was present in his face.

As I grew older, I came to understand that there are people in this world who quit and give up and will offer an excuse at the drop of a hat. I was lucky not to know many of these people until later on in life. I was fortunate to learn from people like George, Rodney, Bill,

John, and so on who showed me what hard work and diligence were all about. I learned a lot about life from those places of employment on Seneca Street and the men and women who worked there. I learned about what it means to persevere and persist and how one's life can actually become happier when perseverance is grounded in faith, hope and love.

The Rule of Persistence

There is a certain quality that all great people possess that enables them to persevere even when things seem to be at their bleakest. This quality of persistence transcends the need to create an excuse to perform any task even when that task is mundane and not profitable or self-fulfilling. This ability to persist manifests itself in individuals who are consistent, productive, punctual, non-judgmental, purposeful, and have grounded their self-awareness in fundamental principles of well-being. Even in the face of doom and sure and uncertain failure, they hang on and don't quit.

In other words, people who persevere, people who persist, people who keep on going simply DO NOT QUIT! They very seldom give in, give up, or give out. Even if they grow tired and weary, they go the extra mile; even if they fall down and suffer from discouragement or disappointments, they pick themselves up, brush themselves off, and start all over again.

This is not to say that they don't get discouraged and that they may not need to stop and refresh or rejuvenate themselves every once in a while, we all need that. But it is to say they do not cave in at the slightest downturn and that they will persist and persevere and give it all that they can.

Do you have goals in your life that you would like to achieve? Are there plans or aspirations or dreams that you want to aspire to? Is there a higher level in life that is leading you onward and upward? Are there things you want to do and places you want to go? If so, then you are like most everyone else, and the key to fulfilling your goals is to plan them out, pursue them, and persist until they are fulfilled.

Usually people who persist have a purpose, and that purpose is more often than not grounded in a deep and abiding affection for someone or something. A love of family, country, work, faith, friends, passions, pets, pleasure, or LIFE! When people have a purpose that is grounded in love, then they are genuinely happy.

An Exercise in Persistence

Read the following story:

THE LITTLE ENGINE THAT COULD
(Watty Piper, 1930)

A little steam engine had a long train of cars to pull. She went along very well till she came to a steep hill. But then, no matter how hard she tried, she could not move the long train of cars. She pulled and she pulled. She puffed and she puffed. She backed and started off again. Choo! Choo! But no! the cars would not go up the hill.

At last she left the train and started up the track alone. Do you think she had stopped working? No, indeed! She was going for help. "Surely I can find someone to help me," she thought. Over the hill and up the track went the little steam engine. Choo, choo! Choo, choo! Choo, choo! Choo!

Pretty soon she saw a big steam engine standing on a side track. He looked very big and strong. Running alongside, she looked up and said: "Will you help me over the hill with my train of cars? It is so long and heavy I can't get it over."

The big steam engine looked down at the little steam engine. The he said: "Don't you see that I am through my day's work? I have been rubbed and scoured ready for my next run. No, I cannot help you,"

The little steam engine was sorry, but she went on, Choo, choo! Choo, choo! Choo, choo! Choo, choo! Soon she came to a second big steam engine standing on a side track. He was puffing and puffing, as if he were tired. "That big steam engine may help me," thought the little steam engine. She ran alongside and asked: "Will you help me bring my train of cars over the hill? It is so long and so heavy that I can't get it over."

The second big steam engine answered: "I have just come in from a long, long run. Don't you see how tired I am? Can't you get some other engine to help you this time? "I'll try," said the little steam engine, and off she went. Choo, choo! Choo, choo! Choo, choo! After a while she came to a little steam engine just like herself. She ran alongside and said: "Will you help me over the hill with my train of cars? It is so long and so heavy that I can't get it over." "Yes, indeed!" said this little steam engine. "I'll be glad to help you, if I can." So the little steam engines started back to where the train of cars had been standing. Both little steam engines went to the head of the train, one behind the other.

Puff, puff! Chug, choo! Off they started! Slowly the cars began to move. Slowly they climbed the steep hill. As they climbed, each little steam engine began to sing:

"I-think-I-can! I-think-I-can! I-think-I-can! I-think-I-can! I-think-I-can! I-think-I-can! I think I can - I think I can - I think I can I think I can--" And they did! Very soon they were over the hill and going down the other side.

Now they were on the plain again; and the little steam engine could pull her train herself. So she thanked the little engine who had come to help her, and said good-bye.

And she went merrily on her way, singing: "I-thought-I-could! I-thought-I-could! I-thought-I-could! I-thought-I-could! I thought I could - I thought I could - I thought I could - I thought I could - I thought I could - I thought I could I thought I could --"

THE END

Source: http://en.wikipedia.org/wiki/The_Little_Engine_That_Could

Now reflect in your own mind on what you think the moral of the story is?

The Persistence Quiz

Rate what you think your Persistence Quotient is by checking the box that best describes your perseverance:

+1	+2	+3	+4	+5
Never Persistent (no stamina)	Seldom Persistent (give up easily)	Somewhat Persistent (hang on until it hurts)	Highly Persistent (hang on longer than most)	Always Persistent (never quit)

My Persistence Score _____

Remember to keep your Persistence Score handy because it will be used at the end of the book when you determine your total Happiness Quotient.

Finally, practice persistence in your life by mindfully becoming aware of events in your life where you can do things without quitting. Literally "go the extra mile" when you feel like giving up. Consciously make an effort to drive yourself outside of your comfort zone and practice persistence. When you do so, you will find that the ultimate result leads to a happy resounding verse of "I knew I could, I knew I could, I knew I could!"

Passion

"Passion is not something to be found. It is something to be expressed. You cannot find your passion by searching for some person, place, interest or activity outside of yourself. Rather, you express your passion within the context of your own life and the world in which you live. Certain things can ignite your passion and help you to more fully express it. Yet the passion itself exists within you and is always there, no matter what happens on the outside. Instead of going in search of your passion, seek to put your passion into everything you do."

-Ralph Marston, 'Expressing Passion,' The Daily Motivator©, June 19, 2003
http://greatday.com

Stories of Passion

One of the most valuable lessons I have learned in life is that if you can follow your passion, you will be the happiest person in the world. In other words, if a person has a passion for art and he becomes a teacher of art, he will most likely be happy. If a person has a passion for helping others and she gravitates her work toward some kind of counseling or social work, she will probably be happy.

The percentage of people who are miserable at their job is astounding, those who are unhappy at what they spend their lives doing is incredible. If only they could somehow tap into their desires, their dreams, their passions, they would much better enjoy getting up each day and facing the world. To implement one's passion in life first takes knowledge of what that passion is, and following one's passion means to find one's purpose.

This lesson was instilled upon me when I was delivering papers to a more than just a few of my customers. Mr. and Mrs. Watson on Mays Avenue were prime examples. Mr. Watson was a music teacher and he had passion for music. I knew this because I could hear him serenading the neighborhood with his trumpet on Saturday mornings when I collected. And sometimes he would be playing a trombone or, if I was really lucky, I would be fortunate enough to hear him play a classical piece on the violin.

The music he played was more than notes played on an instrument; they were melodic voices that spoke to the very heart of the listener. I was more than impressed and more than moved by the passion that came forth from the musical instruments that he played.

And his wife, Vivian was just as passionate as I witnessed when I heard her play the piano on weekday afternoons when I delivered the newspaper. The music coming from the Watson household was so beautiful that more often than not I found myself stopping my delivery schedule and listening with enthralled pleasure at the magnificent pieces that were being performed. This was my first introduction to classical music and I savored it with great joy.

And down the street from the Watson's home, close to the corner there was a man by the name of Johnny, that's all I knew him by, just Johnny. Johnny had a passion for gardening. Not a day went by when the weather was nice that I wouldn't find him out in his garden tending to the carrots or cucumbers or pulling the weeds or doing things that gardeners have to do in order to make their gardens grow.

One time, when it was late in the evening and no one else was around, I happened to hear him talking to his plants. I wasn't sure what he was saying, but it was a strange thing for me to hear; a grown man talking to growing vegetables as if they could hear him. Of course, later on in life I learned that this was his passion, this was his love, this was his life, and he was probably the happiest person on the block because he was following his passion.

There were so many others that I met and learned from on my paper route: Mrs. Vincent who grew flowers, Mrs. Darling who had a passion for taking pictures and loved to show them to me on Saturday mornings when I collected, Mr. Thomas who loved his old cars and was always working on them in his driveway.

Each of these people showed me what it was like to have a passion in your life, to let that passion give you a purpose, and to feel the happiness and peace of mind that naturally follows. I learned to seek my passions and let those passions be my guide to happiness.

The Rule of Passion

There is a deep and abiding necessity that lies within the heart of every person to fulfill some sort of inner need, an inner desire that leads to peace and contentment. There are times when this desire can be satisfied by invoking love upon family or by being with friends or by fellowship and faith. At other times this desire can be felt as an innate calling of the soul to fulfill a longing that cannot be expressed in words. This is your passion and passions come in all sorts of shapes, sizes, and genres. Some people search a lifetime for their passion when it is inside their heart all the time. Your passions are not complex, illusive, esoteric 'somethings' that cannot be touched, but they are a living, real, breathing part of your very heart. Tap into your passions and you have found your very purpose.

A genuine passion is tempered with a desire to do what is good and right. There are good passions and bad passions and sometimes it is necessary to delineate between the two. For example, a person with a passion for intoxicants and mind-altering drugs is not following a passion from the heart. Passions should not be confused with lust because lust usually arises from abusive and wrongful intentions whereas passions arise out of love and a desire to fulfill a dream.

Momentary or passing passions are transitory objects of desire that may lead to temporary happiness. This temporary happiness is built on a weak and shifting foundation and will not withstand the test of time. True passions affect your life and remain a lifetime.

Passions sometimes have to be tempered in the sense that one cannot spend his entire time, energy, or source of income on a particular passion. Mr. and Mrs. Watson loved their music; however, they found other avenues of pursuing life while at the same time enjoying their passion; they taught music, and that was an ideal situation for them. Moderation is an important concept to follow in all aspects of life.

Do you know what your passions are? Are you trying to follow them the best you can in your lifetime? If not, can you do something to bring your passions, your dreams, your desires, into the forefront of your life? If so, you will be a happier and more peaceful person. Following your passions is essential to finding true happiness and peace of mind in life.

<u>An Exercise in Passion</u>

Answer the following questions with honesty and truthfulness. Write your first response, not dwelling on the question or response, but write what first comes to your mind.

1. What you are happiest doing (generally speaking)?
   _____?
2. In defining what you are happiest doing, is it something you can do as a career or job? _____
3. If not, is it something you can do to help you relax? _____
4. List three things you enjoyed doing as a child or young adult:

   a. _____
   b. _____
   c. _____

5. Do you still enjoy doing any of these things at this time in your life? _____
6. List three specific things at this particular stage in your life that bring you the greatest pleasure:

   a. _____
   b. _____
   c. _____
7. Is any one of the three things you listed in No. 6 also listed in No. 1 above? _____
8. Describe your life in 25 words or less _____

   _____
   _____
   _____
   _____
   _____
   _____

9. Describe how you would like your life to be in 25 words or less

_____
_____
_____
_____
_____
_____
_____
_____

10. How close are No. 8 and No. 9 related? _____

_____
_____
_____

11. If they are not very closely related, what would it take to bring them closer together? _____

_____
_____

12. Describe your truest, deepest passion in 25 words or less:

_____
_____
_____
_____
_____
_____
_____

13. Is it possible to fulfill your passion? Yes _____ No _____
14. If 'no' why not; if 'yes' how can you: _____

_____
_____
_____
_____
_____
_____

15. Describe someone you know who lives their passion, what it is, and what he or she does: _____

_____

_____

_____

_____

_____

_____

_____

Now reflect on your answers.

<u>The Passion Quiz</u>

Give yourself +1 point if you answered question No. 12 in the Passion Exercise; 0 points if you did not answer the question; do not go back and answer the question now.   _____

Give yourself +1 point if you answered question No. 13 in the Passion Exercise; 0 points if you did not answer the question; do not go back and answer the question now.   _____

Give yourself +1 point if you answered question No. 14 in the Passion Exercise; 0 points if you did not answer the question; do not go back and answer the question now.   _____

Give yourself +1 point if you answered question No. 15 in the Passion Exercise; 0 points if you did not answer the question; do not go back and answer the question now.   _____

My Passion Score _____

Keep track of your total Passion Score because it will be used at the end of the book.

Finally, if possible fulfill your dreams, follow your passions, and reach your goals by starting small and working your way to becoming the happiest person in the world by following your passion.

Finding your own personal purpose in life is the pathway to happiness and finding your purpose is accentuated by following your passion.

Empathy

"Empathy and a depth of understanding are not just nice things to do. They are powerful strategic tools that will greatly enhance your effectiveness. The better you know and understand the other person's perspective, the more successful you'll be at dealing with that person. Take the time to notice, to consider, to understand, and appreciate the people around you. It is one of the most powerful ways to enhance your own life. You don't have to agree with the other person, just seek to understand. So many problems could be solved or avoided if more people would make the simple effort to understand and appreciate the perspective of others. So many opportunities and possibilities would be greatly enhanced if those involved would seek to better understand each other."

~Ralph Marston, 'The Power of Understanding,' The Daily Motivator©, August 24, 1999 http://greatday.com

Empathy, Mr. Randall, and the Return of David

Recently I asked a group I was conducting, "What is empathy?" One of the participants raised her hand and offered "Empathy is the ability to feel sorry for someone." "Fine, I said, "That's a good start. If that is empathy, then what is sympathy?" She thought a minute but didn't really know what to say. Then another person raised her hand and she said, "Sympathy is feeling sorry for somebody." Looking at the entire group, I said, "That sounds familiar." I then asked, "What then is the difference between empathy and sympathy?"

Finally, one young man raised his hand and added, "Sympathy is feeling sorry for something that happened to someone while empathy is literally putting yourself in another person's shoes and actually feeling their pain." "Well put!" I said, "You hit the nail on the head."

Empathy has an element of understanding added to it. Empathy takes sympathy to a higher level and adds caring and compassion. Empathy is the ability to understand another person's plight in life, whether that be a person who is suffering from pain, a person who is undergoing drug or alcoholic rehabilitation, a person who has lost a loved one, an elderly person who needs compassion, a young teenager who wants to be heard, or just the supermarket cashier who has been on her feet for eight hours straight without a break. To feel real and true empathy for someone else is to understand and appreciate that person; and in understanding people, we understand ourselves better.

As an example of a non-empathetic person from whom I learned empathy, let me return to my Preston Avenue experiences as a newspaper delivery boy and David who was a temporary trainee under my tutelage for about a week.

One sunny afternoon as we were completing our last customers of the day, we met an elderly gentleman who was closing up one of his garages that he owned on Preston Avenue. There were about five garages all connected in a row, all worn and tattered with broken out glass in the overhead doors that were covered over with plywood. The structures themselves were dilapidated old buildings that were decaying and rundown. They looked as old and shabby as their owner. At one time they were probably very magnificent facilities that were a testament to those who parked their automobiles inside to protect them from the elements; but now they were merely places to store excess machines, boxes, materials and junk that no one seemed to have a use for. Now they were merely a storage place where an old man stored his treasures and memories of years gone by.

Mr. Randall was well into his 80s and walked with a cane. I had heard from my father that he once owned a machine shop inside one of the garages and that he could fabricate any tool or metal part that anybody in the area needed. He was a master craftsman in his time, but now his outward appearance gave way to the condition of the machines inside the garages.

I don't know why he was at the garages that day, maybe it was for memories sake, but David and I happened to meet him as he was coming down the loose stone driveway that led to the sidewalk. I greeted him with a smile and asked him how he was doing. We talked a while; he talked about the "old days" when he could fabricate anything for anybody. Then he pulled out two steel ball-bearings from his pocket and showed us how perfectly smooth they were and how they were part of his work.

They were large, about three inches in diameter, and he gave each of us one of them. I remember thinking that these were an old man's treasures and how honored I was to receive this piece handicraft from this once skillful artisan. I could truly empathize with Mr. Randall and the work of his handicraft. I felt a sense of pride and importance in being chosen to be the recipient of what was obviously something he had himself cherished for a long, long time.

I thanked Mr. Randall as I held the ball-bearing in my hand to feel its smoothness and admired its shininess. I then turned to David to see if he had any words of thanksgiving to offer to our generous friend when David did something that I could not believe. Taking the ball-bearing in his right hand, he jerked his arm back and then flung the ball-bearing across the creek bed that was across the one-way street, saying out loud, "Let's see how far this baby will fly…" And in an instant, it was gone. In disbelief, I looked at Mr. Randall and I could see a small tear running down his cheek. He wiped it with the back of his hand, turned around and silently walked away from the both of us.

I didn't know what to say to David. In utter disbelief, I remember saying something to the effect, "How could you do that?" And his only reply was, "Do what?" And there it was, one of the most valuable lessons I have learned in my life; the lesson of empathy, or the lack thereof.

What a valuable lesson I learned from that experience. There are those in life who have absolutely no clue about empathy, caring, understanding, compassion, or the feelings of others; those who simply do not care. But I also learned that the world is made up of those who do have a caring nature, an empathetic heart, and a kind and considerate spirit; and it is those who maintain this quality of empathy that are more at peace with themselves and happier with the world and those around them.

The Rule of Empathy

The ability to transcend one's own feelings and emotional ownership and place oneself in the very soul of someone who is feeling pain, loneliness, dejection, depression, or in need of comfort, compassion, understanding, companionship, or a caring attitude is to epitomize the very core of empathy to its fullest extent. To have an empathetic nature is to feel the goodness of all humankind and surpass the test of understanding in all its forms. The opposite of empathy can be defined as lack of character. Empathy leads to inner peace and inner peace leads to happiness and the splendor of great joy.

The lesson learned from David's lack of empathy was a lesson that followed me throughout my life. I often think back and wonder whatever happened to poor David. I wonder if he was able to feel empathy for anything or anyone at any point in his life. I wonder if he is happy or if he is alone somewhere, eternally destined to live in a lonely world.

Like all of the other ingredients that have been mentioned, empathy can be acquired but it takes a conscientious attitude and practice. If you do not have an empathetic nature or a caring heart that comes naturally, that does not mean that you cannot conscientiously think of these things and make an effort to practice empathy in your daily life.

Empathy is not meant to be something that is evasive or hard to follow but something that can be consciously applied, but in doing so it must be appreciated and understood as a resource for helping others. In helping others it becomes a stepping stone for ourselves to peace, contentment and happiness.

Exercises in Empathy

Exercise A

For this exercise, visit a facility where there are a lot of different people from different walks of life; a mall, a supermarket, an airport, a bus depot, or a park. Or you can do the exercise while waiting at the doctor's or dentist's office or some other office where other people are waiting. Finally, the best place of all to do the exercise is by visiting a hospital or nursing home and sitting in the waiting area and watching the different people who go by. This is an exercise in watching people and empathizing with their situations.

1. Pick out someone in the 'crowd' of the place you have chosen who is suffering or having a difficulty or problem in some way. It could be a person who is walking with a walker or crutches, a mother trying to quiet her baby, a young man in a wheel chair, someone who has been hurt, and so on.

Try to place yourself in that person's position. Have you ever been in that type of situation yourself so that you know exactly how that person feels? If so, then you know what that person is going through and how he or she feels.

Make a conscientious effort to mindfully think about that person's feelings and what it would be like to be that person. What would you feel like? Mindfully say to yourself, "I have been there, I know what you are going through."

2. Pick out someone in the 'crowd' or place you have chosen who appears to be impatient and irritated for some reason. It could be someone in line at a supermarket or someone annoyed because they have to wait too long for an appointment, and so on.

Try to place yourself in that person's position. Have you ever been in that type of situation yourself so that you know exactly how that person feels? If so, then you know what that person is going through and how he or she feels.

Make a conscientious effort to mindfully think about that person's feelings and what it would be like to be that person. What would you feel like? Mindfully say to yourself, "I have been there, I know what you are going through."

3. Pick out someone in the 'crowd' or place you have chosen who appears to be happy and smiling and filled with great joy, someone who is obviously having a wonderful day and doesn't seem to let anything bother them.

Try to place yourself in that person's position. Have you ever been in that type of situation yourself so that you know exactly how that person feels? If so, then you know what that person is going through and how he or she feels.

Make a conscientious effort to mindfully think about that person's feelings and what it would be like to be that person. What would you feel like? Mindfully say to yourself, "I have been there, I know what you are going through."

Exercise B

Go to your newspaper and read an obituary of someone who recently passed away. Go to the list of surviving relatives. Think about one of the relatives and how they feel about the loss of their loved one.

Try to place yourself in that person's position. Have you ever lost a loved one yourself? If so, then you know how that person feels and the grief they are experiencing.

Make a conscientious effort to mindfully think about the feelings of the relatives. Think about their loss and how they feel. Mindfully say to yourself, "I have been there, I know what you are going through."

Note that this exercise may bring up sad memories of your own losses and cause you to feel sadness and grief for your own loss. If this is the case, this is okay because we all experience losses in our lives. I can empathize with you because as I write this, memories of my own loss of my mother and father come to my mind. Grief of a loved one is universal. The fact that we cared for them and loved them is why we feel grief. The sadness of the loss of a loved one can be overcome with the joy of the memories and the knowledge and understanding that their spirit lives on forever.

The Empathy Quiz

In situation A1 rate your situational empathetic quotient. Were you able to "feel" the pain of the person who was suffering or had a problem? How empathetic were you? Check the box that corresponds to your empathetic nature:

+0	+1	+2	+3	+4
no empathy at all	a little empathy	some empathy	empathetic	very empathetic

In situation A2 rate your situational empathetic quotient. Were you able to "feel" the pain of the person who was irritated or annoyed? How empathetic were you?

+0	+1	+2	+3	+4
no empathy at all	a little empathy	some empathy	empathetic	very empathetic

In situation A3 rate your situational empathetic quotient. Were you able to "feel" the joy of someone who was happy? How empathetic were you?

+0	+1	+2	+3	+4
no empathy at all	a little empathy	some empathy	empathetic	very empathetic

In situation B rate your situational empathetic quotient. Were you able to "feel" the grief of someone who lost a loved one? How empathetic were you?

+0	+1	+2	+3	+4
no empathy at all	a little empathy	some empathy	empathetic	very empathetic

Now add your scores together to get your total Empathy Quotient:

My Empathy Score _____

Remember to keep your score so that we can add them together at the end with all your other scores.

Finally, practice empathy every chance you get. Take the exercises in the book a step further and create your own scenarios where you can practice empathy. Try it on family members, friends, church members, even strangers. Before long you will discover that an empathetic nature leads to an understanding heart which cultivates itself with love and happiness ensues.

Serenity

"Take a deep breath, and calm your thoughts. Rise above the noise and confusion of the day, to a place that is peaceful and serene. Let go, for a moment, of the need to judge, to analyze, to criticize and to strategize. Let go, for a moment, and experience how beautiful it is to just be. All is well in this moment. It's perfectly fine to simply enjoy it for a while. Your problems, your dramas, your possessions are all very small compared to who you are. Take just a little while to remember that. Give yourself a refreshing respite of peace, of calm serenity. Then take it with you in all you do".

~Ralph Marston, 'Serene Respite,' The Daily Motivator©, November 18, 2003 http://greatday.com

"There is no need to give up your serenity for the sake of getting something accomplished. In fact, accomplishment comes more surely when your efforts are calm and your spirit is peaceful. Consider how very much more you can get done when your energy is not being sapped away by a frenzied mind. True serenity is not the absence of action, but rather action with integrity, confidence and a steadfastness of purpose".

~Ralph Marston, 'Respond with Serenity,' The Daily Motivator©, December 19, 2003 http://greatday.com

The Serenity of Mrs. Stewart

I had many customers who were my favorites and one of my favorite people to visit was Mrs. Stewart who lived on William Street. She lived by herself in a very modest house on a very modest lot. There was nothing fancy about her home, nothing fancy about her appearance, and nothing fancy about her lifestyle. She was a widow, probably in her early 80s and she had no close family that lived nearby, no friends, and no visitors; in fact, I think my Saturday morning visits to collect were sometimes the only visitors she would have for the entire week.

On weekdays she would very often greet me at the front door. She would be waiting as I got off my bicycle to take the paper and place it inside the front screen. Mrs. Stewart would always have a smile and invite me in to sit and talk a little bit and I never said no. We would always chat about unimportant things, but things that were important to her. She had a cat that kept her company and she would like to tell me about how mischievous he had been that particular day or how he had gotten into a fight with a neighboring cat and got scratched up. She always had something to talk about.

There was something very calming and serene about Mrs. Stewart; something that comes from age or wisdom. I could hear it in her voice, I could see it in her eyes, and I could feel it in her spirit. She would talk about her family from long ago and how she raised six children who are all grown now and moved away. She would talk about her many years of working for the telephone company as an operator. She would talk about her deceased husband and how much they enjoyed life together.

Her conversations were stories that were laden with passion and a sense of serenity. Whenever I took five or ten minutes to visit with

Mrs. Stewart it was like the entire world had stopped and I didn't have a care in the world. There could be a hurricane or an earthquake outside and I don't think it would have interrupted our visit. She had that special quality of capturing the moment and solidifying it with tranquility and peace. Whenever I talked with Mrs. Stewart, I always came away feeling a little bit better about myself, a little bit happier.

In reflecting on the many "Mrs. Stewart's" I have met in my lifetime since my early childhood experience and the lessons I have learned from them; I have come to the conclusion that they all have many good characteristics, but one in particular stands out as being a major virtue. They all seem to have a sense of serenity about them that transcends the chaotic world around them. This component of serenity seems to be an essential element in those who have tapped into unconditional happiness in their lives.

Serene people are those who have a natural feeling of tranquility about them. It can almost be described as an aura of sacredness as well as a positive attitude.   I find myself gravitating toward people like that because of their positive nature and good spirit. In aligning my life to such people, I have found that my principles, my beliefs, my lifestyle, my world view, my credo, my very nature are reinforced and bolstered by that beautiful first stanza of the Serenity Prayer by Richard Niebuhr that was referred to earlier in the section on the Rule of Acceptance.

God grant me the SERENITY to accept the things I cannot change; COURAGE to change the things I can; and the WISDOM to know the difference…

The Rule of Serenity

Avoid negative and callous people who have impure motives and navigate your life around those who are pure of heart, have a positive attitude, and generate a spirit of tranquility and peace. In your own life, practice a sense of calmness and a demeanor of stillness and harmony. When you need to, step back from the 'maddening crowd' and enjoy life. Stop and smell the sweet aroma of happiness. Serenity is a state of mind that allows you to accept the things you cannot change and to savor the splendor of its simplicity.

Life is filled with the "Mrs. Stewarts" of the world who will naturally generate a sense of harmony, calmness, and stillness. Seek them out, they are there. You probably won't find them in bars or dance studios or night clubs; you may not find them on Facebook or Twitter; but you will find them if you open your mind and heart to the message that they preach and practice. It is a message of faith, hope, and love that is grounded in peace, tranquility, and serenity.

One of the members of my groups that I conduct recently shared a story when we were talking about serenity. She said that she was at home, cooking dinner for her and her small children. She said the television was blaring, the phone started to ring, the doorbell rang, the baby was crying, her six-year old was screaming, and the pot on the stove was boiling over, and she just couldn't take it anymore. So she stopped!

She turned the television set off; she turned off the stove, turned off the telephone, held her baby in her harms and sat down with her six-year old and just closed her eyes and enjoyed the moment. For just a few short minutes, she was able to feel a peaceful calmness, and that serenity that enveloped her seemed to rejuvenate her and give her the energy she needed to make it through the rest of the day.

There were others in my group that said that they found great peace and serenity in prayer and meditation and others said they found it in surrendering to their Higher Power. Everyone agreed that when they were able to find peace and serenity it made them a happier person.

Have you ever been in a situation in your life when you just needed to step back and rest and feel the calmness of the moment? Have you ever felt the need to just stop for a moment, reset your weary eyes and rest, relax, and rejuvenate? Are you able to do that? It takes practice, like all of the rules mentioned in this book.

Quiet your life, still your fears, calm your anxieties, and lessen your stress and you will know the joy of using the Rule of Serenity as a way to happiness. In the midst of chaos and confusion and calamity, seek out serenity and you will find happiness.

Exercises in Serenity

Exercise A

Make a list of all of the things in your life that are causing your life to be less than serene. Call this list "Stress Factors in My Life" and know that these are the things that cause anxiety, apprehension, and angst.

Take your list of "Stress Factors" and analyze it carefully. See if you can categorize the factors that lead to your stress. Are they financial worries, are they relationships, are they employment related, are they grief related, and so on.

Reflect on each item on your list and how you have handled these in your life.

Exercise B

Reread the first stanza of the *Serenity Prayer* by Richard Niebuhr

God grant me the SERENITY to accept the things I cannot change; COURAGE to change the things I can; and the WISDOM to know the difference…

1. Make a list of some of the things you cannot change in your life that cause you anxiety.

2. Make a list of the things you can change in your life that cause you anxiety.

Note: This list may be the same list that you used in exercise A above but you may now begin to refine it.

Do you have the courage to change the items listed in B2 above? Reflect on your answer.

Exercise C

1. What causes you to have peace, tranquility and serenity?

Make a list of those things. Are they things that are easily obtainable or things you can do readily? Are they things you can do more often? Are they honorable, good, and pure things that you are proud of?

2. How do you prevent yourself from "burn out"? What do you do to relax? Do you have any hobbies or things you like to do to keep occupied?

Make a list of these things. Are they things you can do more often? Are they things you should be doing more often?

The Serenity Quiz

On a scale of 0 - 10 rate your *serenity level* with +0 being no peace or serenity and +10 being complete peacefulness, tranquility, and serenity in your life.

+0	+1	+2	+3	+4	+5	+6	+7	+8	+9	+10

no serenity → → → → → → → → → → → → → complete serenity

serenity level _____

On a scale of 0 - 10 rate your *stress level* with +0 being a life with absolutely no stress at all and +10 being a life filled with complete stress, anxiety, and debilitating pressures.

+0	+1	+2	+3	+4	+5	+6	+7	+8	+9	+10

no stress → → → → → → → → → → → → → complete stress

stress level _____

Now subtract your *stress level* from your *serenity level* to determine your Serenity Quotient:

serenity level _____

(minus) -*stress level* _____

temporary Serenity Score _____

If your score is a negative number (your stress is higher than your serenity) then record a +0. If your score is <u>below</u> +10, then add +2 points to your score if you answered Exercise C2 with a "yes" regarding the question, "Do you have any hobbies?" If you have a hobby or something to prevent "burn out" then add +2 points to your

Serenity Score; however, your total Serenity Score <u>cannot exceed</u> +10 points.

My Serenity Score _____

Remember to keep your score handy until the last section of the book to determine your Happiness Quotient.

Finally, practice the Rule of Serenity whenever and wherever you can; as often as you can, and enjoy the peaceful solitude of the calmness of your life. Read books on how to relax, take retreats, learn how to incorporate the Rule of Serenity into your life and you will be a healthier and happier person.

Niceness

"You will never regret genuine kindness. You will never regret making the most of whatever is available to you. Though it may be painful at the time, you will never regret being truthful. And you will never regret giving your best effort to whatever task is at hand. You will never regret the time you spend with those you love. And whether or not it is appreciated, you will never regret giving a helping hand to those in need."

~Ralph Marston, 'Never Regret,' The Daily Motivator©, January 21, 2002 http://greatday.com

"It's easy to act with kindness and understanding toward those who have been kind to you. Yet the real power of kindness comes when you give it even to those who don't deserve it. Reacting with cruelty in response to cruelty only drags down everyone involved. With kindness, you have the opportunity to lift up yourself and others. Being kind does not mean allowing others to take advantage of you. On the contrary, your kindness can give you the positive, undeniable power to make sure that everyone's best interests are served."

~Ralph Marston, 'The Power of Kindness,' The Daily Motivator©, July 17, 2002 http://greatday.com

The Epitome of Niceness

Kindness, compassion, gentleness, kindheartedness, benevolence, thoughtfulness, consideration, selflessness, amiability, congeniality, friendliness, geniality, and cordiality; these are all synonyms for the word "niceness." What a powerful word. Have you ever met anyone with these qualities? If you have, don't you consider them quite remarkable people?

Niceness is an important and integral part of the total formula for a happy, productive, peaceful and content life. Without the quality of niceness or kindness, life seems a little bit more dreary and little bit more ordinary. Add niceness and you are adding an element of sweetness that takes life to a higher level.

In my lifetime I have met quite a few people who can fit the description of niceness, and those whom I have met have left a lasting impression upon me and inspired me to be a little kinder, a little nicer, and to perform as many acts of kindness as I possibly can. As a rule, people who are nicer are happier.

There was one particular person I met who happened to be a customer on my paper route, a man who changed my life forever. He worked in one of the car dealerships on Seneca Street where I delivered the newspaper; it was the Pontiac and Cadillac garage that was located at the far end of Seneca Street next to the Gulf gas station. I would visit the garage every day to deliver the paper and every day this gentleman would be there.

He was a hard working man who was always at the garage. If he wasn't in the showroom demonstrating a car to a customer, then he was out in the garage checking on a customer's automobile or in the part's department getting parts that were ordered for another customer.

Sometimes on weekday afternoons he would be talking to a family about a car that they might be interested in, and if he was he would stop what he was doing and take time to wave to me or say hello and ask me how I was doing.

Sometimes he would be in the middle of a big sale, a new Cadillac with a very important client, and yet he would excuse himself and come to meet me at the doorway to pick up the paper and talk for a little bit.

No matter where I saw him or when I saw him, he always had a good natured grin, a genuine smile on his face. He was well known for his smile and friendly nature and had the reputation as being the most "honest car salesman in the county." He had earned many awards for his salesmanship as was attested to by the numerous plaques and trophies displayed in his small office at the dealership.

His entire countenance displayed kindliness and an openness and all of those words used in the first paragraph that denote niceness. And what was even more important was that his niceness was genuine, it came from the heart. I learned a great deal from this man in seeing him at work and in other places as well because he was more than a customer on my paper route he was also my father, Charles F. McCormick. I think of the many things my dad taught me and the many things that I learned from him and one of the most endearing virtues is this quality of niceness or kindness that he portrayed so well in his actions.

There were times when I had seen him so tired after working a twelve-hour day and yet he would offer to do something for someone, pick up groceries for them or take them to the doctor. After he had passed away I became aware of stories from complete strangers who told me how he had given them money when they were down and out or how he had helped them in a time of need. People still remember his big kind smile, his good natured attitude, and his overall niceness.

Even though we didn't have a lot of possessions and we couldn't afford a lot of things that other families had, we had a great deal of love and happiness which resulted from my father's attitude toward life. He was a very happy man, a very content man; and I think my mother and my three brothers and I grew up happy because of that happiness that he instilled in our home.

My father taught me that without the quality of niceness you suffer the consequences of a very lonely life and that niceness breeds niceness. He was a very wise man who never went to college but had more knowledge than people I know who have PhD's. He knew about life and that one of the fundamental principles of life was to live life being as happy and content and peaceful as possible. He understood that this could be achieved through a gentle peace of mind and that peace of mind comes by practicing the quality of niceness.

The Rule of Niceness

In every situation in life, in every opportunity that arises, even in the face of disenchantment and discouragement, be nice to others. Niceness produces niceness. The nicer you are to others, ultimately, the nicer they will be to you. Niceness and kindness are synonymous with happiness. When in doubt, practice niceness; when in fear, practice niceness; when in pain, practice niceness; for practicing niceness will lead to an inner peace and harmony that brings forth happiness.

Have you ever had a sugar cookie without sugar? If you are used to salt and pepper, have you ever tried a meal without using it? Many people like different spices, cinnamon on toast, chili powder, vanilla, and mint; one of my favorite spices is Oregano. Ask any great chef and they will tell you that cooking without spices is not cooking at all. Food without spice is tasteless food.

Niceness is the spice of life and a life without niceness is weak, ordinary, insipid, mediocre, and can be downright mean and nasty. What would the world be if the quality of niceness were taken away? What if there was not one individual in the world that was kind or thoughtful? I wonder how long the human species would endure. Not very long, I am sure. We only go through this world once, why not make it a little happier through our acts of kindness toward one another, our own personal commitment to being nice by following the Rule of Niceness.

Exercises in Niceness

Exercise A

Go to your local newspapers or a recent magazine or if you prefer, go to your computer and find a story that has to do with someone doing something nice for someone else. Read the story and reflect on the events surrounding the circumstances. Place yourself in the shoes of the person who received the act of kindness. How do you think that person felt? Now place yourself in the shoes of the person performing the act of kindness. How do you feel?

Exercise B

Make a list of ten things you can do that to make things a little nicer in your home environment, in your relationship, in your school, in your job, or for yourself. Reflect on this list. Is there any reason why you cannot do any of the things on the list in order to make things nicer?

Exercise C

List three *nice* people whom you know in your life. Next to their name, list three qualities for each person. In looking at the list of qualities, is there any quality that all three people have? If so, what qualities are they? Write them down and reflect on them. Are they qualities that you have in your own life? Are they qualities that you can aspire to? Why did you select the three people whom you selected?

The Niceness Quiz

For each of the following items that you can answer "yes" to, check off the box to the right. This is an opportunity for you to earn "extra" points that you may have lost in other categories.

In the last month, did you ever:	(yes) +1
Visit a sick friend or a hospital or nursing home.	
Call someone who was lonely or someone unexpectedly.	
Offer to help someone with homework, a project, or housework.	
Give someone a ride somewhere.	
Mow someone's lawn or shovel snow for someone.	
Donate money or time to a charitable organization.	
Compliment someone even though you didn't like them.	
Give a hug to anyone for any reason at all.	
Volunteer in any capacity (church, school, work, etc.).	
Thank the cashier at the supermarket with a genuine smile.	
Write a thank you note to anyone for any reason at all.	
Leave an extra big tip for a waitress or waiter even though the service wasn't that great.	

Life Rules: A Manual to Attain Happiness

Tell someone that you have forgiven them.	
Buy lunch or dinner for a friend or acquaintance.	
Let the driver on your right go before you when you both stop at a stop sign at the same time.	
Donate food to a food pantry or food drive	
Send a gift anonymously to a friend or charitable organization.	
Try to cheer someone up who was depressed.	
Bake something (cookies or bread or cake) for someone.	
Remember someone who has lost a love done with a phone call, card, plant, or food.	
Make someone feel good.	
Buy something for somebody because they didn't have enough money.	
Invite someone who is alone to share a meal with you or go out to coffee or lunch.	
Tell someone how much they are appreciated.	
Take care of a pet for someone who was away.	
Water plants or watch a house for someone who was away.	
Take someone to the movies or to a show or concert.	
Take someone to church or a doctor's appointment.	

Now total up the number of "yes" responses that you have checked in all of the responses above _____

Because niceness is such an important category you should be able to earn "extra credit," so your total may be greater than the amount that is allowed for the Happiness Quotient to equal 100 at the end of the book. Therefore, if your score is *more than* +18 you can only record +18 points as your Niceness Quotient. The fact is though; you still had the opportunity to earn extra points by responding to 28 questions. This will all make sense at the end of the book.

My Niceness Score _____ (+18 is the highest score)

Keep this score along with your other scores as we will be putting them all together at the end of the book to determine your total Happiness Quotient.

For now, let's see how "nice" you are:

your score:	you probably:
+18 above	are a very nice person
13 – 17	are a nice person
8 – 12	are nice some of the time
4 –7	need improvement
0 – 3	need "nice" training

Finally, as always, practice makes perfect. Practice the Rules of Niceness in your life every opportunity that you get and you will be a happier person.

Putting it All Together

"Try as you might, you cannot make yourself happy with what you do not have. When you wait for happiness or make it conditional, it never does materialize. Happiness is a choice, not a result. Nothing will make you happy until you choose to be happy. No person will make you happy unless you decide to be happy. Your happiness will not come to you. It can only come from you. Happiness is what you are, not what you have. It depends solely upon your own attitude. You can be happy no matter what your circumstances might be. You can never get happy. You can always be happy. Lift your own self-imposed restrictions on happiness. Count your many blessings, and be happy. Spread your happiness and it will grow."

~-Ralph Marston, 'Happiness,' The Daily Motivator©, September 22, 1998
http://greatday.com

And so, we come to the point now where we can put all of these nine Rules together into some sort of order and see what we come up with. Before we do that, there are a couple of things I want to review with you in order to see if you can come up with the point this last section of this text book is trying to convey.

First, let me list the nine Rules of Life for peace, contentment and happiness that we discussed. Here they are in the order they were presented in the book:

The Rule of Simplicity

The Rule of Humility

The Rule of Acceptance

The Rule of Integrity

The Rule of Persistence

The Rule of Passion

The Rule of Empathy

The Rule of Serenity

The Rule of Niceness

While each Rule could stand by itself, it is important that you consider the nine rules together because they formulate something very important, one of the key subject matters of this book that has been mentioned over and over again.

To better understand what I am talking about, remember that at the end of each section, you took a small quiz and determined your own individual score for each of the Rules. For example, you have your own personal Empathy Score, your own Niceness Score, your own Integrity Score, and so on.

The rules were presented in somewhat of a random order, but now is the time to put them all together. Now is the time to fill in your scores on the following score sheet to determine your Happiness Quotient. In order to do this, you may have to go back and see what your score was for each Rule, or you may write your scores on a piece of paper and transfer them here. I have taken the order of presentation from the book and put them in a different order here. You will see why in a minute.

Please record your scores for each sectional quiz that you completed:

My Humility Score   _____ (possible +6)

My Acceptance Score   _____ (possible +15)

My Persistence Score   _____ (possible +5)

My Passion Score   _____ (possible +4)

My Integrity Score   _____ (possible +8)

My Niceness Score   _____ (possible +18)

My Empathy Score   _____ (possible +16)

My Simplicity Score   _____ (possible +18)

My Serenity Score   _____ (possible +10)

    My Happiness Score   _____ (possible +100)

Before we discuss your score, do you notice anything about the arrangement of the scores listed above?

Do you see the *point* of why all of these Rules work together?

Can you see what I am talking about? Does it make sense now?

If not, take the first letter of each of the Rules. Do you see it now or do I have to *spell* it out for you? Okay, I will:

> *The Rule of **H**umility*

> *The Rule of **A**cceptance*

> *The Rule of **P**ersistence*

> *The Rule of **P**assion*

> *The Rule of **I**ntegrity*

> *The Rule of **N**iceness*

> *The Rule of **E**mpathy*

> *The Rule of **S**implicity*

> *The Rule of **S**erenity*

Put them all together and what do they spell: *h-a-p-p-i-n-e-s-s*

As stated above, while each one can stand alone, each one is also an integral part of the whole. In order to achieve total, lasting, and unconditional happiness, it is important to follow all of the rules the best you can.

As far as your total Happiness Score or Happiness Quotient is concerned, how did you do? Did you score in the 90th percentile or 80th percentile? Or perhaps you were you at the other end of the spectrum near the 70 percent range?

I'm not going to place the scores on a scale and tell you whether or not you are happy because only you know that for sure. No book, course, psychologist, psychiatrist, counselor, minister, or anyone or anything can tell you that. Only you know whether or not you are happy.

The purpose of this book is to offer you a guide, a manual, a handbook on how to achieve some things in your life that may help you find a little inner peace, contentment, fulfillment, joy, pleasure, bliss, satisfaction, and ultimately happiness in your life. It is my firm belief that you can accomplish this if you follow the nine rules listed in this book.

Finally, here is a review of the nine Rules of Life that lead to happiness. Try to learn them and practice them daily in your life.

H

The Rule of Humility

When in the course of daily events you have any opportunity to learn from someone, grasp that moment with full abandon and savor those times like treasures more valuable than gold. Never underestimate the power of humility for in humbleness you will earn the respect of every person your path of life encounters. Humility is the secret to inner acceptance which leads to great peace of mind, and peace of mind leads to happiness.

A

The Rule of Acceptance

There are events and circumstances in life that cannot be changed or altered because they are out of our control. Acceptance of this fact of life relieves the mind and frees the spirit to accomplish great tasks and to ground our lives with an inner peace beyond description. The acceptance of who we are leads to an awareness of what we can do which in turn creates a euphoric sensation in our lives that generates a genuine and lasting purpose in life. Acceptance is a major component to happiness, satisfaction, peace, and joy in all of life's endeavors.

P

The Rule of Persistence

There is a certain quality that all great people possess that enables them to persevere even when things seem to be at their bleakest. This quality of persistence transcends the need to create an excuse to perform any task even when that task is mundane and not profitable or self-fulfilling. This ability to persist manifests itself in individuals who are consistent, productive, punctual, non-judgmental, purposeful, and have grounded their self-awareness in fundamental principles of well-being. Even in the face of doom and sure and uncertain failure, they hang on and don't quit.

P

The Rule of Passion

There is a deep and abiding necessity that lies within the heart of every person to fulfill some sort of inner need, an inner desire that leads to peace and contentment. There are times when this desire can be satisfied by invoking love upon family or by being with friends or by fellowship and faith. At other times this desire can be felt as an innate calling of the soul to fulfill a longing that cannot be expressed in words. This is your passion and passions come in all sorts of shapes, sizes, and genre. Some people search a lifetime for their passion when it is inside their heart all the time. Your passions are not complex, illusive, esoteric 'somethings' that cannot be touched, but they are a living, real, breathing part of your very heart. Tap into your passions and you have found your very purpose.

I

The Rule of Integrity

On the journey of life you will meet many people. Some will be as honest as the day is long while others will take advantage of you and seek to connive and manipulate every aspect of your being. You must be on guard and discern in your heart those who are pure and those who have motives that are untrustworthy. Concerning your own self, integrity is the highest form of self respect and inner awareness that leads to true and lasting contentment, happiness and blissfulness. The adage, "To thine own self be true," means to live with integrity in your heart, your mind, your soul, your self, and every facet of your life. Integrity is more than a state of mind; it is a state of being, a state of existence, a state of daily accomplishment that manifests itself in word and in deed; what you say and what you do.

N

The Rule of Niceness

In every situation in life, in every opportunity that arises, even in the face of disenchantment and discouragement, be nice to others. Niceness produces niceness. The nicer you are to others, ultimately, the nicer they will be to you. Niceness and kindness are synonymous with happiness. When in doubt, practice niceness; when in fear, practice niceness; when in pain, practice niceness; for practicing niceness will lead to an inner peace and harmony that brings forth happiness.

E

The Rule of Empathy

The ability to transcend one's own feelings and emotional ownership and place oneself in the very soul of someone who is feeling pain, loneliness, dejection, depression, or in need of comfort, compassion, understanding, companionship, or a caring attitude is to epitomize the very core of empathy to its fullest extent. To have an empathetic nature is to feel the goodness of all humankind and surpass the test of understanding in all its forms. The opposite of empathy can be defined as lack of character. Empathy leads to inner peace and inner peace leads to happiness and the splendor of great joy.

S

The Rule of Simplicity

Consciously eliminate regrets, frustrations, failures, and guilt of the past. Do not add anxious worrisome thoughts about what may or may not happen tomorrow. As best you can, concentrate on the moment you are in and fulfill that moment with good thoughts and positive affirmations. Weigh in your mind the things you need as opposed to the things that you want in every aspect of your life. And realize that to downsize is to utilize the best of what you already have.

S

The Rule of Serenity

Avoid negative and callous people who have impure motives and navigate your life around those who are pure of heart, have a positive attitude, and generate a spirit of tranquility and peace. In your own life, practice a sense of calmness and a demeanor of stillness and harmony. When you need to, step back from the 'maddening crowd' and enjoy life. Stop and smell the sweet aroma of happiness. Serenity is a state of mind that allows you to accept the things you cannot change and to savor the splendor of its simplicity.

Whatever your endeavors in life, may you come to realize that true happiness and peace begin from within and that your life is a beautiful gift that is meant to be enjoyed and appreciated. Live life to its fullest by appreciating the splendor of its beauty.

There is one more quote I would like to use to recapitulate the essence of what we have been talking about in this book; how to achieve happiness, inner peace, tranquility, and contentment in life. This is the poem called *Desiderata*, which means "things desired" as written by Max Ehrmann in 1927. Pay particular attention to the very last line as it speaks highly of what this book is all about:

Desiderata
Max Ehrmann 1927

Go placidly amidst the noise and haste, and remember what peace there may be in silence. As far as possible without surrender be on good terms with all persons. Speak your truth quietly and clearly; and listen to others, even the dull and the ignorant; they too have their story.

Avoid loud and aggressive persons, they are vexations to the spirit. If you compare yourself with others, you may become vain or bitter; for always there will be greater and lesser persons than yourself.

Enjoy your achievements as well as your plans. Keep interested in your own career, however humble; it is a real possession in the changing fortunes of time.

Exercise caution in your business affairs; for the world is full of trickery. But let this not blind you to what virtue there is; many persons strive for high ideals; and everywhere life is full of heroism.

Be yourself. Especially, do not feign affection. Neither be cynical about love; for in the face of all aridity and disenchantment it is as perennial as the grass.

Take kindly the counsel of the years, gracefully surrendering the things of youth. Nurture strength of spirit to shield you in sudden misfortune. But do not distress yourself with dark imaginings. Many fears are born of fatigue and loneliness.

Beyond a wholesome discipline, be gentle with yourself. You are a child of the universe, no less than the trees and the stars; you have a right to be here.

And whether or not it is clear to you, no doubt the universe is unfolding as it should. Therefore be at peace with God, whatever you conceive Him to be, and whatever your labors and aspirations, in the noisy confusion of life keep peace with your soul. With all its sham, drudgery, and broken dreams, it is still a beautiful world. Be cheerful.

Strive to be happy.

Source: http://en.wikipedia.org/wiki/Desiderata

About the Author

Robert W. McCormick has been involved in education, ministry, or chaplaincy for most of his life. He has over 40 years of teaching experience, most of which has been at the college level as a full time professor. Included in his teaching experience are more than ten years of online education. For the last five years he has been the director of online education and distance learning for a private college, also teaching two to three classes per semester. Deacon and Professor McCormick has earned two master's degrees, one in theology and the other in education.

As an educator at the college level, he has authored or co-authored two major textbooks, two handbooks, two workbooks, a glossary/dictionary, and teacher's manuals to accompany the textbooks. All of the books are published by a major publishing house and are currently being used by many colleges. In addition, he has created tutorial software relating to the textbook material and markets and sells the software through another publishing company.

As a permanent deacon, the author is an ordained clergyman and assigned to a parish with parish responsibilities. His duties also include a chaplain's position at a hospital and nursing home.

As a chaplain he has conducted workshops and spirituality groups for clients who are in alcohol and drug rehabilitation programs, bereavement groups, and elderly day care programs and church related groups.

The author also reads and writes extensively on the topic of angels and is currently working on two books dealing with angels. He has written numerous magazine articles about the angels and has given a number of workshops that deal with angels.

Deacon McCormick lives in a small upstate New York community with his wife and has three grown children and six grandchildren. He can be reached at the following email address: bob@infoblvd.net

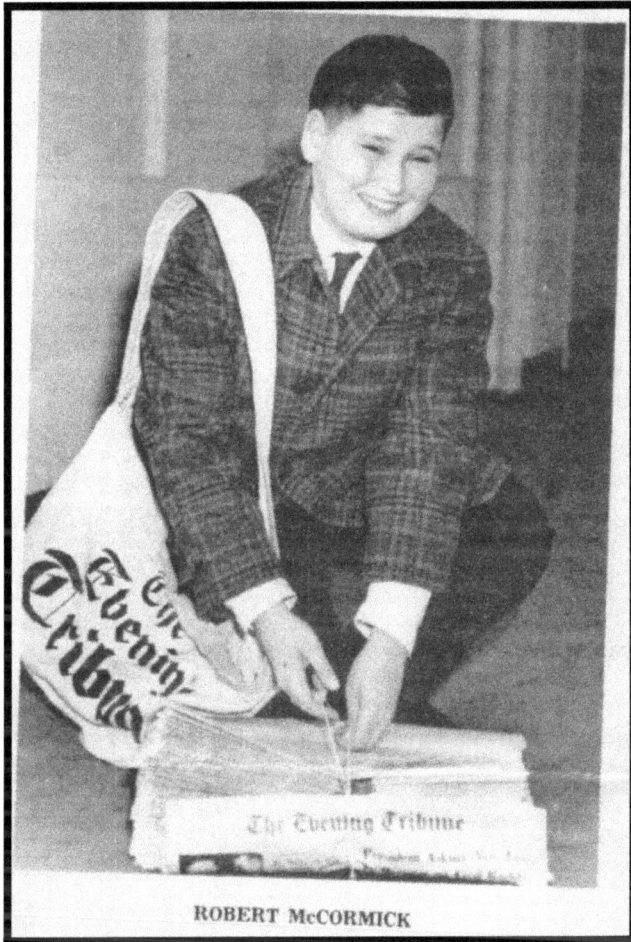

ROBERT McCORMICK

February, 1963

Carrier Boy of the Year

Deacon Robert W. McCormick

Life Rules: A Manual to Attain Happiness